"*The Miracle of Health* is not just a reminder, but also a constant guide to keep exercising. It offers a program for all of us to get and stay healthy. Uche and Kary not only give us the guide, but provide ongoing cheerleading and inspiration to stay the course. *The Miracle of Health* is for everyone who wants to live better and longer."
> —*Dr John Ratey, M.D., author of* Spark, *clinical associate professor of psychiatry, Harvard Medical School*

"Uche and Kary are walking, talking examples of living a healthy lifestyle that is enriching, honoring the connection between the physical, emotional, and spiritual. I recommend *The Miracle of Health* to everyone. It is an inspiration to all of us."
> —*Cathy Jameson, Ph.D., founder and CEO, Jameson Management, Inc., Oklahoma*

"Finally! A health and wellness book for real people that offers real solutions, not a false, temporary fix. This dynamic duo inspires us with timeless wisdom that makes active living fun."
> —*Judith Wright, author of* The Soft Addiction Solution *and* The One Decision, *Chicago*

"Uche and Kary are the picture of perfect health. They possess the unbridled passion and unlimited energy needed to whip any couch potato into shape."
> —*Thor Diakow, associate producer,* "*Breakfast Television,*" *CityTV, Vancouver*

"Each time I turned to Kary and Uche's writings to get refocused and remotivated, their spirit and enthusiasm live in their words and inspire me to get back on the path. I ran two half-marathons during cancer treatment, and felt they were with me every step of the way."
> —*Rita Smith, director of communications, Health Canada, Ottawa*

"Uche and Kary will help you get fit, be fit, and live fit."
> —*Mark Victor Hansen, coauthor of* Chicken Soup for the Soul, *California*

"*The Miracle of Health* is a powerful, inspiring read. If you're looking for motivation and an action plan, this book is for you!"
—*Dr. Melissa Hershberg, M.D., author of the best-seller,*
The Hershberg Diet, *Toronto*

"Kary and Uche—in their uniquely high-energy, personal, and motivating way—convince us that the true miracle of *The Miracle of Health* is that it lies within each of us to live a healthier, more active life. They coach us to unleash our innate ability and build upon our strengths."
—*Kelly Murumets, CEO, ParticipACTION Canada*

"The most inspiring health and fitness book in the past 10 years. It's impossible to read it and not be motivated for change."
—*Dr. Steve Rasner, D.D.S., New Jersey*

"A truly inspirational guide to achieving optimal health and vitality. . . . *The Miracle of Health* reminds us that within each of us lies the potential for greatness and lifelong vibrant health and wellness."
—*Dr. Nadine Cyr, naturopathic doctor, Toronto*

"*The Miracle of Health* provides clear guidance and ignites fresh inspiration to reach your personal, professional, and spiritual goals. Kary and Uche are the catalysts who will help you transform powerful reasons into meaningful results. This book not only changes you physically, but stimulates you mentally and makes you believe that nothing is impossible!"
—*Almira Cuizon, regional director, Guess Canada*

"Kary and Uche have already helped motivate and change the lives of thousands of people around the world. Let them help you become more aware and motivate you with *The Miracle of Health*."
—*Dr. Glenn Bailey, chiropractor, Winnipeg*

THE
MIRACLE OF
HEALTH

THE
MIRACLE OF
HEALTH

SIMPLE SOLUTIONS, EXTRAORDINARY RESULTS

DR. UCHE AND KARY ODIATU

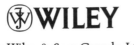

John Wiley & Sons Canada, Ltd.

National Library of Canada Cataloguing in Publication Data

Odiatu, Uche
   The miracle of health : simple solutions, extraordinary results / Uche Odiatu, Kary Odiatu.

Includes bibliographical references.
ISBN 978-0-470-15661-2

   1. Health.   2. Physical fitness.   I. Odiatu, Kary   II. Title.
RA776.O343 2008   613   C2008-904935-7

Production Credits
Cover design: Ian Koo, Mike Chan
Interior text design: Adrian So
Typesetting: Thomson Digital
Printer: Quebecor World–Fairfield

John Wiley & Sons Canada, Ltd.
6045 Freemont Blvd.
Mississauga, Ontario
L5R 4J3

Printed in the United States

1 2 3 4 5 QW 12 11 10 09 08

Contents

Acknowledgments

First, thanks to everyone who has attended our live programs, acted on their health goals, and shared their renewed inspiration and commitment with the people in their lives. We enjoy receiving your e-mails and hearing how our strategies have assisted you on your path to wellness. We feel privileged and honored that you have found such value in our message.

Thank you to the media who have invited us to entertain and educate the viewers and listeners. You help us fulfill our goal to help others take action.

Special thanks to the team at John Wiley & Sons who have encouraged and supported us in our quest to write *The Miracle of Health*, a timeless guide for personal health transformation. We are especially grateful to Leah Fairbank for her patience and guidance.

We are inspired by the entire Genuine Health team for their passion and commitment to supporting people with their health needs. Their dedication to research and development is incredible. A special thank you to Sam Graci, Stewart Brown, Lisa Chisholm, Beth Potter, and Letelle LeClair.

Our greatest thanks is to our families and friends, who provide us with our very own powerful reasons to pursue our passion. Relationships are the true texture and juice of life. We feel blessed to have such amazing people in our lives.

And a huge heartfelt thanks to *you*, the reader. We respect, admire, and are grateful for your investment of time and energy.

Make life magical!

In health there is freedom. Health is the first of all liberties.
—Henri Frederic Amiel

Introduction

WARNING: Some side effects of reading this book may include:

- An energized personality

- Healthy relationship with yourself and others

- Compliments on your muscle tone

- Feeling comfortable in your skin

- Smiling during physical activity

- Glowing, vibrant skin

- Resilience to stress and depression

- Freedom from aches, pains, and stiffness

- Enhanced brain function and memory

- Decreased risk of dementia, Parkinson's, and Alzheimer's

- Increased bone density and fewer breaks

- Reduced risk of heart attack, stroke, diabetes, and cancer

- Strength to maintain your independent lifestyle

- Confidence to participate in new activities

- Feeling refreshed from deep sleep

- More checkmarks on your to-do list

- Promotions at work due to your increased productivity

- More *Chi*, *Prana*, or life-force energy

- Renewed goals and dreams

- Anticipation for your active retirement plans

- Inspired family, friends, and colleagues

Sounds a little too good to be true, doesn't it? That is why we called this book *The Miracle of Health*. The preceding list isn't just another empty promise; it is the reality you can expect after implementing the lifestyle changes we are about to share. It's amazing how fast it can happen. And you don't need to change your entire life today. Too many changes done at once will set you up for failure. The journey of a thousand miles begins with a single step—start even one new healthy lifestyle habit and you will get the ball rolling. It's like a snowball. It starts off small, but with concentrated effort, that snowball will grow exponentially. And the science is in: Your lifestyle choices are *key* to enhancing the quality of your life. We're not talking about small, insignificant benefits. We mean miraculous changes to every one of the 120 trillion cells in your body!

What Is a "Miracle" Anyway?

If you change the way you look at things, the things you look at change.
—Wayne Dyer

Can you imagine an amazing life filled with energy? Can you picture yourself enjoying your reflection in the mirror? Or would that require a miracle at this point?

You deserve to look and feel good! But to be a person who enjoys boundless energy and freedom from aches and pains, you need to do certain things each day. It's like a recipe. If you follow the directions, you will enjoy the same result. Remember the last time you leafed through a cookbook? And you stopped to linger on the picture of something that looked delicious? The author guaranteed that if you followed the recipe, you too would be able to make the same scrumptious-looking food. Okay, let's change the example: this is, after all, a health book, not a cookbook. If you followed a healthy person around for one week, took notes, and then replicated what he or she did, you would move toward creating the miracle of your own toned, healthy body.

We once heard Marianne Williamson, author of *The Age of Miracles*, say that a miracle can be viewed simply as a change in perception, and that changes in perception can happen over time or instantaneously. Quantum theorists say our consciousness influences the environment that surrounds us. And consciousness is influenced by perception, which means that changes in perception can alter the world around you. Whether you want to look at this from a spiritual point of view, or a scientific point of view—we think it is miraculous that your world can be altered when you see things in a new light.

This book will open your eyes to the power of your intention; by teaching you how to focus on positive perceptions, better food choices, and daily movement, it will put you on a collision course with health miracles!

It all starts with a simple decision and action steps toward its fulfillment or, as our friend and co-author of *Chicken Soup for the Soul*, Mark Victor Hansen says, "Ful-thrillment."

> ### *Health Miracle*
>
> **Numerous studies make the connection between weight loss and psychological well-being. Once a person takes action and begins to lose excess weight, they will experience benefits beyond the physical.**

The Obesity Epidemic

Poor diet and physical inactivity is second only to smoking in lifestyle factors contributing to the nation's top killers, including Coronary Artery Disease (CAD). Inactive people have a 45% greater chance of developing CAD.
—American Heart Association, Centers for Disease Control

There are more fat-free products, fitness facilities, certified personal trainers, fitness magazines, diet centers, plastic surgeons, and fat burners than ever before, yet we are the heaviest we have ever been, and we are *still* packing on the pounds. Our sedentary lifestyles and poor diets have caught up with us. It is well established in scientific research that being overweight or obese is directly related to a low-energy expenditure lifestyle combined with a high-calorie diet.

> *Some futurists are predicting that at this rate, 95 percent of North America will be overweight by 2030.*

Obesity increases the risk of a number of diseases, including cardiovascular disease; type 2 diabetes; osteoarthritis; post-menopausal breast cancer; and cancer of the uterus, colon, kidney, and esophagus. All of these often lead to premature disability and death. *Fat* is considered the new tobacco by The Heart and Stroke Foundation in Canada. They report that the number of overweight and obese people has risen by 60 percent since the 1970s and the number of deaths directly related to obesity has doubled in the last 15 years. We have read statistics from other sources that say 30 percent of U.S. children are overweight, almost six times the number in the 1980s. Type 2 diabetes among children is at an all-time high.

CNN doesn't remind us about the tragedy of approximately 2,000 people dying per day of heart disease, but we all hear about the latest shark attack. Something is wrong with this picture! Isn't it ironic that your chances of dying from heart disease are about one in two, and your chances of dying from a shark attack are about one in 300 million?

Health Miracle

In his January 2004 update, the Director of the U.S. National Cancer Institute stated: "It is abundantly clear that regular physical activity can reduce the risk of colon cancer by half, and can also reduce the risk of breast cancer among obese postmenopausal women."

North America Needs a Miracle!

You can't leave footprints in the sands of time if you are sitting on your butt. And who wants to leave buttprints in the sands of time?
—Bob Mowad

This book will inspire you to choose the top foods eaten by the healthiest, longest-lived people on the planet. And if you really want to know what the best diets are, we have found them! We will tell you the secrets of people who have lost weight and kept it off. If you are interested in doing this without going to a gym, turn to Chapter 6, "Goodbye Fat, Hello Fitness" and enjoy new strategies from the NEAT lab at the Mayo Clinic to increase your daily metabolic expenditure. For those of you up to the challenge, we have included some of our favorite workouts (all designed with the latest research on maximizing your exercise time) in Chapter 7.

In Chapter 6 we have also revealed the revolutionary research into a chemical that researchers refer to as "Miracle-Gro" for the brain. Through exercise, you can exponentially increase this chemical and experience the benefits of a healthier brain—better memory, focus, concentration, and decision making.

One of the most important chapters in the book, Chapter 8, will take away every excuse you have ever had for not exercising or choosing better foods. Once you say "goodbye" to your excuses, you can say "hello" to the good life. No one will ever call you a procrastinator again!

Throughout the book, we have also included the activities, stories, and health miracle highlights that inspire our seminar, television, and radio audiences to take daily action toward creating their own health miracles. Now we want to share this incredible information with you!

You will find that underlining and circling information can start the ball rolling. All of the quotes in the text were carefully selected to enhance the material you are reading. If one touches your heart or hits home with you, write it down in your journal or stick it on your fridge. Write in the margins of the book, highlight material, and turn down the corners of the pages. Go ahead, mark it up—you paid for it! We do this to our favorite books. *The Miracle of Health* is not a short-term ticket to losing weight and squeezing into your wedding dress or business suit. You will find it is so much more!

In the Zen tradition, sages talk of the beginner's mind, the ability to have an open mind when you are looking at new information. Miracles can take place when open your mind by simply asking yourself: "How can this information serve me?" This process is called *cognitive restructuring*. Just by reading highly charged material, changes may occur. You'll see. This stuff sort of sneaks up on you.

This book was written with powerful intention. We feel that we were inspired to help millions of people transcend their slow, sedentary lives. We know why we wrote this book. By reading it until the end, you will fulfill your end of the bargain. The payoff will be days filled with energy and a lifetime of abundant health and vitality.

We have searched high and low—from our own personal experiences, the best books on health, the proven success principles from the top authors, the greatest minds to walk the planet, to the longest-lived people on Earth—for the best advice to simplify your own journey to better health. Or, if you are already on your way, we will help you kick it up a notch!

The information in *The Miracle of Health* will empower you to bridge the gap from knowing to doing. It will take the facts from your brain and imbed them in your heart. Emotion leads to motion, so fuel up your muscles and get your butt off the couch!

Health Miracle

In May 2008, The American College of Sports Medicine trademarked the slogan: "Exercise is medicine," and called on every medical professional to assess and review each patient's physical activity and progress at each visit.

Chapter 1

Every moment is a second chance to turn it all around.
—Eminem (rapper), from the autobiographical
movie *8 Mile*

What Is Your Powerful Reason?

It might seem unusual to quote Eminem in a book called *The Miracle of Health*, but this isn't your average health book. There is no better time to choose health than right now! All of your power is in the present moment. As Eminem implies, every moment offers the opportunity to make a change. And we have uncovered a secret that can help you make changes and get over roadblocks to great health: You need to have a *powerful reason* that will inspire you for a lifetime!

You see, most people attempt to get in shape for short-term, ego-bound reasons. They want to lose weight so desperately they make statements like, "Even if it's gonna kill me!" And why?

"Summer is four weeks away."
"My fortieth birthday is coming up."
"My best friend just lost 10 pounds."
"I'm going on vacation."
"It's my high school reunion this spring."
"I just made a bet with my co-worker."
"I just lost a bet with my co-worker."

Losing weight is still the number-one reason for most people to start a program and our "quick-fix" society is inundated by a plethora of products and supplements "guaranteed" to work fast. Sure, you might get some results, but statistics show that less than 5 percent of all dieters experience long-term success. Most of us know people who have thrown themselves into a Herculean workout and starvation diet to get into that small dress or suit. Those intense efforts may bring immediate results—that's what makes them attractive—but they aren't maintainable. It's like cramming all night for the big exam. Sure, you might pass, but the knowledge is soon lost. Short-term, ego-driven goals do not lead to long-lasting habits or results. You need long-term, powerful reasons that will inspire a lifetime of great health.

Health Miracle

You control more than 70 percent of how well and how long you live. By the time you reach fifty, your lifestyle dictates 80 percent of how you age; the rest is controlled by inherited genetics.

—Dr. Mehmet Oz and Dr. Michael Roizen

What Is a Powerful Reason?

A powerful reason is one that will nag you to get up and do something; it is a constant reminder of where you would like to be in life. A powerful reason inspires you to move, even when you don't feel like it because it brings up the emotions that inspire action. Esther Hicks, in *The Law of Attraction*, says that you need to think of these inner emotions as a guiding force. If you listen to your inner guide, you will make decisions that move you closer toward how you want to look and feel.

We have to acknowledge that not every powerful reason necessarily comes from a positive source. We have spoken to people who have made major changes in their lives because a significant other called them "fat," or because they suffered a severe health crisis. Ego-bound reasons and negative circumstances can sometimes lead to positive changes. The important thing is that once you take matters into your own hands and get started, you will eventually find new, powerful reasons that will be much more positive—reasons that will serve you for life!

Seminar Attendee's Story

During a break in one of our spa getaway seminars, a lady approached and told us that she finally reached rock-bottom the day she overheard her former boss refer to her as a "wide load." She vowed on that day to lose the excess weight that she had been carrying for years. She used her anger at his comment to get started—and never looked back. She stood before us, slim and glowing. She now has the powerful reason of enjoying her newfound life-force energy. I'm sure she would thank that man if she ran into him today.

Here are some of our favorite powerful reasons:

1. For Family

The energy we expend in nurturing must always be replenished with self-care and self-development if we are to mother optimally.
   —Dr. Christiane Northrup

Your family and their health may be at the top of your priority list. The problem is that most caregivers forget to take care of themselves. Why do we think we are serving our loved ones when we neglect our own health? Research shows that inactive parents have a very low chance of having active children.

The bottom line is that all of the relationships in your life are a reflection of the most important one: the one you have with yourself. The best way to take care of the people around you is to care for yourself first. Recall the last time you were on an airplane and the flight attendant announced, "In the event of an emergency, the oxygen masks will lower from the ceiling. Place the mask around your face first. Then you may assist others."

2. For Love

Success in your fitness endeavors will spill over into all other areas of your life, especially your relationships. When you exercise, your body produces feel-good hormones, the same hormones you experienced when you first met that special someone. As anyone who has ever been in a long-term relationship knows, production of those hormones subsides over the years. Why not take advantage of the hormonal workout response and get your loved one to the gym or out for a walk? If you are active together, you will associate all those feel-good hormones with each other. Being fit also means feeling better, and the better you feel, the more available you will be for the people in your life. Have you ever tried to listen to a loved one talk about a tough day when you had a sore lower back?

3. To Be a Role Model

Actions speak louder than words. Whether it is at home, at work, or at play, you are probably a role model for someone in your life. People admire and respect those who have a healthy discipline with their exercise and nutrition. A friend who made some lifestyle changes and lost 18 pounds recently told us that everyone at work was suddenly interested in her lunch choices. This boosted her confidence and gave her more encouragement to stick to her healthy eating plan. So start a new health habit today and watch the people around you stand up and take notice.

4. To Be a More Effective Leader

It is a well-known fact that U.S. presidents make time for physical activity. Many top Fortune 500 companies that have incorporated on-site fitness facilities for their employees report extraordinary increases in productivity and decreases in sick leaves. We uncovered so many benefits related to leadership that we developed a seminar called "Fit to Lead," and it is one of our most popular programs! In Chapter 6, we have included more exciting research about this topic.

5. Because Your Body Is Your Temple

Every man is the builder of a temple called his body.
—Henry David Thoreau

The body is an incredible machine, a powerhouse, nature's masterpiece, and a scientific marvel. Each action is a miracle in itself: a wound healing, food digesting, your incredible heart beating, your lungs breathing (an average of 21,000 times a day), your cells tingling with enough electricity to cause a lightning bolt. Your body is a gift. You received one body at birth that can function well into the eighth and ninth decades of life, so treat it well and chances are, you will experience a long, healthy, fulfilling life.

Health Miracle

Your heart is only the size of your fist, and yet it beats about 86,000 times per day and sends out 2,000 gallons of blood through blood vessels. These vessels would circle the Earth twice if they were placed end to end.

6. For Your Mental Health

Sickness is not what the body is for.
    —Helen Schucman and William Thetford

If having a well-functioning body is not one of your worries, then how about your brain? Excess weight can be detrimental to brain function. It is one of the biggest contributors to Alzheimer's and, according to John Ratey's revolutionary book, *Spark*, about exercise and the human brain, "Simply being overweight doubles the chances of developing dementia, and if we factor in high blood pressure and high cholesterol—symptoms that often come along with obesity—the risk increases sixfold."

7. To Be an Active, Independent Older Adult

The biggest problem in health care today is that we don't take care of our-selves.
    —David Chilton, author and motivational speaker

Our good friend and mentor, nutritional researcher Sam Graci, speaks of quality of life in your elder years. He believes that aging should be an enjoyable process with a quick, painless passing at the twilight of your life. In his book, *The Path to Phenomenal Health*, Sam tells of his 94-year-old father, who began his own health renovation at 85 years of age only after a major health crisis. He went on to experience the best decade in his life: "Papa Joe taught us how a Wise Elder should exquisitely expire. I held him in my arms while he shouted 'I am ready, I am ready—I want to go home now,' elegantly passing beyond the shores of life."

There is no better insurance for graceful aging than good nutrition and exercise. In fact, there is so much evidence that your lifestyle can determine how long you live and how well you live that we decided to devote an entire chapter to the subject. Fast-forward to Chapter 9 if you think this may be your powerful reason to *take action*.

8. To Create Some Leverage

What does it take to get people moving and eating more vegetables? Often it's a crisis or a tragedy. Some people hit rock-bottom before they come to the realization that their current practices aren't serving them.

And, all too often, we hear of someone starting an exercise program after a quadruple bypass. Spiritual guru Marianne Williamson once said that if you have not faced any tragedies by the time you hit 50, then get ready! The human experience comes with its trials and tribulations. That is why we want you to equip yourself for the unexpected curveballs life will throw your way. We strongly advocate that, if for no other reason than to avoid a health tragedy, you start taking care of yourself now. It is all about preparation or, as Dr. Mehmet Oz says, "Stack the odds in your favor!"

We faced a time of great despair in our own lives with the birth of our first child in 2004. We were the healthiest people, with the most positive outlooks, joyfully expecting our first child, with all the dreams of new parents. We expected to enjoy our new son and all of the pleasures that come with watching our child develop and grow. But this was not to be for us.

Jordan was born with a rare, neurological condition. We lived at The Hospital for Sick Children for the first five weeks of his life, enduring test after test and trying to cope with the news that our son would not live a normal life span; that he would not grow and develop like other children; that he would not be able to eat food by mouth; and that he would suffer from terrible seizures. We were informed that he would never walk, talk, or even sit on his own. One doctor told us he would probably never even smile. We were told that he would have a very short life span and that we could not take him home from the hospital unless we agreed to have a G-tube inserted into his stomach. He was unable to eat orally due to lack of coordination with his swallowing, which could allow food and liquid particles into his lungs (aspiration) and lead to pneumonia and other serious chest problems. Jordan was labelled medically fragile, needing complex, 24-hour care. In order to take him home, we would have to learn how to feed him through this tube and administer the many medications he would require for seizures and other problems like reflux, poor bowel movements, and the constant threat of aspiration.

We finally agreed to the G-tube procedure and Jordan was released from the hospital. Nursing care was set up in our home, and thus began the daily schedule of medications, chest physiotherapy, occupational therapy, and daunting feedings (every G-tube feed could take anywhere from one to two hours).

Kary's Experience

I felt like I was in a sinking ship, with no escape. I was so over-whelmed with grief that I rarely left the house for fear that I would see other mothers out with their "normal" babies. All my dreams of mommy-baby classes, and play dates were replaced with the reality of frequent medical visits, evaluations, and sleepless nights as I constantly checked to make sure that Jordan was properly positioned to facilitate easier breathing and have less chance of aspiration from the severe reflux.

Finally, I reached out for a lifeline and headed to the gym for my first workout since giving birth. I couldn't bear the thought of returning to the same gym where everyone had seen me happily progress through my otherwise normal and healthy pregnancy, so we joined a new facility and I was relieved to be among strangers who would not be rushing over to ask about the baby.

As I entered the door, a sense of comfort immediately enveloped me: the gym had always been the one place I could go to relieve stress, forget about all my problems and, for a brief moment in time, escape into my own meditation in motion. From the first rep to the final stretch, I allowed myself to be completely in the present moment. With every deep breath, I could feel a lightening of the cloud that was constantly hanging over my head. I felt good for the first time in weeks. On the way home, my eyes welled up with gratitude for the fact that I was strong and healthy because I knew this would enable me to cope with the cards we had been dealt.

I actually came home with a smile on my face that day. I knew that everything would be okay as long as I continued to take care of myself. Within weeks, the boy that would never grow up started smiling back at us. It was a miracle for our family.

What Is Your Powerful Reason?

The most compelling reason for you to *take action* might be in this chapter. You may discover it on the very last page of the book, or you may find it somewhere else in your life. You will know when it happens because your pulse will quicken as you realize what you have to do and why you must *take action* at that moment. When this happens, we want you to pause for a minute. For that exact moment will mark a turning point for you. It is another chance for a renewed way of living. Once you uncover your very own personal, strong, emotionally charged reasons, you will be compelled to exercise consistently and enjoy it, eat nutritious foods in appropriate amounts and savor them, create an amazing environment for the important people in your life and truly feel fulfilled, and enjoy the aging process without fear.

Karla's Powerful Reason

For the last four weeks, I have taken the steps to live a healthier more active lifestyle and I am now seeing some results and feel so much better already. After hearing you speak, I know that I am doing this for more important reasons than looking good in those tight jeans. This is for my health and for my baby boy. I lost my mom to cancer when I was 18 (she was only 46) and she never saw her grandson. Cancer has taken out the last two generations of my family and I don't want to be the third!

Health Miracle Activities

1. Close your eyes and imagine all of the important people in your life. Now fast-forward your life and imagine the impact a chronic, degenerative disease will have on your loved ones if you do not make any changes to your current nutrition and fitness.

2. Write down your powerful reasons for wanting to change your lifestyle. Do you want to be a great role model for your loved ones, for your colleagues, or for your clients? Do you envision yourself as living a life of independence, experiencing the gift of aging gracefully and actively? Do you want to be a more energetic husband, wife, or parent? Do you see yourself as a powerful, inspiring leader? Write down your own powerful reasons to take action:

   1. _____
      _____

2. _____
   _____

3. _____
   _____

With the preceding desires acknowledged and recorded, you have started a magical process. By placing your interests in writing, you have focused your attention and set time-tested forces in motion. Remember the words of Yul Brynner as the pharaoh in Cecil DeMille's epic film *The Ten Commandments*: "So let it be written, so let it be done!"

Whenever you pick up *The Miracle of Health*, come back to this place and reread your powerful reasons. Doing so will reaffirm your resolve and help you become more aware of the information and strategies that will enable you to achieve your goals.

You are the only one who cares passionately about your health!
   —Kary Odiatu

Chapter 2

If you don't exercise your body, then your muscles begin to constrict. And if you don't exercise your mind, then your attitudes begin to constrict. And nothing constricts your life experiences like the constriction of your thoughts. It limits your possibilities, and it limits your joy.
    —Marianne Williamson

The Inner Game of Health

Every person is what he is because of the dominating thoughts which he permits to occupy his mind.
   —Napolean Hill, author of *Think and Grow Rich*

Everything can be taken from a person but one thing: to choose one's attitude in any given set of circumstances—to choose one's way.
   —Viktor Frankl, concentration camp survivor

When most people think of health, they focus on the physical aspects, yet our physical expression of health is a direct reflection of our inner attitudes toward eating, exercising, and healthy lifestyle activities. Your attitude affects your health blueprint; it is who you are and it is always showing up. It is how you think, speak, and ultimately act. Attitude is defined in the *Oxford Dictionary* as: "A person's way of interpreting or reacting to his or her world." Your attitude is like the set of your sail. With a great attitude, you can sail through life. With a poor attitude, you could very likely end up dashed on the rocks with little left but a single broken oar. Okay, let's not get too dramatic! If your attitude toward a healthy lifestyle is not good, rest assured that like the set of a sail, it can be adjusted to take you to a new destination, a place where you will enjoy an energetic, flexible, and powerful body. This chapter explores how your attitude toward health can open the door to miracles or slam it in your face.

A Winner's Attitude

You have to believe in yourself when no one else does. That's what makes you a winner.

—Venus Williams, champion tennis pro

Having an achiever's attitude is akin to having mastery over your mind. Throughout history, people's thoughts played a large role in the quality of their lives. Milton wrote, "The mind is its own place, and in itself, can make a Heaven of Hell, a Hell of Heaven." Shakespeare once said, "There is nothing good or bad, but thinking makes it so." Emerson reported, "Great men are those who see that thoughts rule the world." Do we need to go on? Okay, one more. Proverbs 23:7 says, "As a man thinketh in his heart, so he is."

It is important to remember that the mechanism that changes the set of your sail can become rusted and loose. We know how easy it is to let your mind wander and dwell on negative thoughts that drift from worry to fear. Being afraid can lead to immobilization and, when that happens, progress can begin to seem impossible. In order to keep the mind well lubricated and strong, we have to take care of it, just like any other vital system in our bodies. If we want to strengthen our muscles, we must progressively add resistance. Similarly, the mind can do incredible things if challenged. By managing the mind, we can attract anything we want into our lives. We call this life management. Does this point intrigue you? If it does, then read on.

Uche's Story

When I graduated from dental school and entered private practice, one of my early dental mentors told me that it would be impossible to maintain my workout regime with a busy practice. I allowed these words to permeate my thoughts and I began to exercise a little less and eat a little more. And over an eight-year period, my health and fitness level decreased dramatically.

This one-time competitive athlete now had love handles. I didn't do any aerobic exercise, so I would become winded with the slightest exertion. My pant size grew, and I would make excuses for wearing oversized clothing: "Designer wear is supposed to be loose."

The sad part was I knew deep inside that this was not how I had planned on feeling. I knew I did not like the way I looked. But I still had the belief that it was impossible to have above-average fitness as a busy professional. I was now living out the consequences of my belief system. It was not that I had intended to look and feel unhealthy. It was just that my attitude of expecting less of myself because of a preconceived notion had penetrated my everyday thinking and behavior.

I was sick and tired of feeling sick and tired. So I took action. I rented a stationary bike so that I could do some aerobic exercise at home where it was more convenient for my busy schedule. I rented instead of buying because I knew that at least 80 percent of home gym equipment sits unused. I was determined not to be part of the 80 percent—so I put the bike in my living room, right in front of the TV. I felt better immediately. Within a few days, I also renewed my commitment to resistance training and headed back to the gym. I couldn't believe that I had left it for so long.

Health Miracle

Being an optimist could be one of the best attitudes for your health. A study at the Mayo Clinic found that the mortality rate of pessimists was 19 percent higher than that of optimists. The good news is that Martin Seligman, author of *Learned Optimism*, says optimism is a skill that can be learned.

The Health Mindset

If you think in positive terms you get positive results—if you think in negative terms you get negative results.
   —William James, American psychologist and philosopher

Have you ever taken the time to reflect on your health mindset? Most people look at exercise negatively: they use it as punishment for overeating; they see it as an obligation, as time consuming, or as boring; and many think of it as pain. And don't worry: if you struggle with food, you're not the only one! The words "fast" and "convenient" have replaced "home-cooked" and "nutritious." As a result, many people are confused about what qualities to look for in food. People have lost sight of the fact that every bite you eat is fuel for your cells. You wouldn't buy the cheapest materials to build your dream home, so why purchase frozen dinners and frequent the drive-thru on a regular basis?

It is time to break free of old habits and ways of thinking. Start making positive associations with a healthier lifestyle. Try thinking of your exercise program as a break from your stressful workday, or as your chance to have time to yourself. It might also be a great opportunity to meet new friends! Focus on the energy and mood boost that you will get from your program and remind yourself that with every step you take or weight you lift, you are immediately improving the quality of your life!

Health Miracle

Positive thinking stimulates excellent health by raising your youth hormone (DHEA or dehydroepiandrosterone), your energy neurotransmitter (dopamine), and your mood-control neurotransmitter (serotonin).

What Are Your Values?

Fix your eyes on what you can do, not back on what you cannot change.
  —Tom Clancy, author

Financial guru Suzie Orman deals with the inner game of wealth. She starts her consultations with discussions about a person's beliefs and attitudes toward money, asking questions about how the person was raised and how his or her role models talked and felt about money. She knows that identifying and working on these values affects her client's financial future more than any advice she gives about the latest "hot stock."

Our early role models play a part in shaping the attitudes we have toward many areas in life, including health and fitness. If you grew up in a household where physical fitness was a priority, you probably find it easy to include some form of fitness in your life. If physical fitness was not a part of your upbringing, you may find it challenging to incorporate it into your present schedule. No matter how you were brought up, the important thing is that you take charge of your health by assuming responsibility for it now.

Your behaviors will change only when you link them directly to important values. Many of you reading this book may never have associated your values with health. While you read *The Miracle of Health*, we are sure that you will see a direct link between your health and the things that are important to you.

Do you value your marriage? Do you value your freedom? Do you value your independence? Your health has a direct impact on all of these areas. If you value financial success, you'll be interested to know research shows that your fitness level has a direct impact on your productivity at home and at work. In the 2006 issue of *Smart Money Magazine*, an article titled "How to Make a Million" listed health as the number-one strategy in a five-part action plan to increase wealth. Or, if you value your family, you will want to read on to discover how families that play together, stay together.

Seminar Attendee's Story

> One of our attendees had been aggressively saving for retirement with her husband for many years. After listening to us speak and participating in a powerful closed eye visualization about her health and her future, she realized that she would never live long enough to enjoy her savings if she didn't take immediate action. She proclaimed: "My lifestyle sucks. I need to take better care of myself so that some other broad is not spending that retirement money!"

Stinking Thinking!

All that we are is a result of what we have thought.
   —Buddha

Did you know each of us has approximately 60,000 thoughts a day? Hardly a waking second goes by without you having a thought! Picture your mind as a factory in which the conveyor belt continuously moves thoughts past the viewing area. Sadly, research shows that approximately 80 percent of thoughts are negative or self-deprecating. John Izzo, in *The Five Secrets You Must Discover Before You Die*, likens the incessant self-talk to a hypnotic trance. We hear people repeating:

"I am destined to stay out of shape." "I hate the way I look." "I am not good at sports." You get the picture? A factory that uses shoddy production practices manufactures poor-quality goods; your mind is no different.

Deepak Chopra, author of the *Magical Mind, Magical Body* audio-cassette series, reports that every thought has a physiological effect on our bodies. Every cell in your body is eavesdropping on your internal and external dialogue. Just by thinking about a negative incident from your past, you not only relive it in your mind, your body also experiences a response as well. The body does not, in fact, distinguish a real event from a memory. Can you imagine the impact that years of replaying old scenarios will have on your entire body?

Health Miracle

Every thought has a physiological effect on our body. Candace Pert, Ph.D., in her landmark book, *Molecules of Emotion*, unveiled a new scientific understanding of the mind/body connection: The power of our minds and our feelings can affect our health and well-being.

Worry and Your Body

Therefore do not worry about tomorrow, for tomorrow will worry about itself. Each day has enough trouble of its own.
     —Matthew 6:34

Like negative thinking, worry can also take its toll on your body. Where do you think the phrase, "I worried myself sick" came from? Many people dump toxic waste into their bodies by way of their thoughts.

Brian Tracy, a peak human-performance specialist, talked about some intriguing research about worrying: He found that only 8 percent of all your worries are justified and only half of those worries, about 4 percent, are in your control. In other words, 96 percent of our worries are needless. According to the love doctor, Leo Buscaglia "Worry never robs tomorrow of its sorrow, it only saps today of its joy." Worry will ultimately drain the mind and body of energy.

Lisa's Story

Lisa had always prided herself on having a curvy figure and good looks, yet she had never really worried about her weight and had never been an exerciser or athlete. She married young and had two children in her early twenties. Her weight started to creep up after having the first baby and after the second, she found herself out of shape and extremely overweight at 5 feet 5 inches and 180 pounds.

What turned it around? One day while at the grocery store, Lisa's son, who had just begun to talk, proudly proclaimed, "Mommy's got a round bum." That statement and the frustration of having nowhere to shop for attractive clothing was enough to make Lisa take action.

She started walking and doing some light resistance training in her home with dumbbells and a bench. She decreased her portion sizes, reduced her intake of unhealthy fats, and started reading books and magazines about health. Within a few years, Lisa had lost all of the weight and managed to maintain a lifestyle that still included wine on the weekends and the ability to indulge at parties and other fun events.

Now, nearing 40, and finding that it is very easy to add 5 pounds if she isn't strict with her nutrition, Lisa still struggles with accepting herself and finds herself looking at other women her age who are very fit. She often thinks: "If only I could be a little more disciplined."

She would love to just accept that it is okay for her to have a few more curves and that there are more important things to worry about in your forties than the size of your pants. She would like to just be happy with the size 6 that is easily maintainable, but constantly finds herself yearning to get back into the size 4.

"I'm trying to accept my current body, but I'm scared that if I totally get beyond the physical aspect of myself, that I might lose the motivation to stay fit. I don't want to gain back all of the weight I lost years ago. . . ."

Body Image

One day you will look back at a picture of yourself when you were in your 20s or 30s and say: "and I was unhappy with that . . . ?"
—Marianne Williamson, author

We think that people have it backwards: we try so hard to impress others, yet fail to be impressed with ourselves. If we could learn how to be happy in our own bodies and comfortable with ourselves, then other people's opinions wouldn't matter so much.

Our first impressions are often based solely on physical appearance. The old adage, "You don't get a second chance to make a first impression" holds true! Sure, people shouldn't judge each other on appearance alone. But, the fact is, people see the outside first and look at the inside later. And the media plays a huge part in how we look at ourselves and others. We are bombarded with countless images of "perfection" on television and in movies. But this is not reality; it is just a representation of the popular culture, a false yardstick by which we learn to judge ourselves and others. In fact, some of you may be sitting there right now saying, "If only I were 10 pounds lighter or 2 inches taller. If only my legs were longer or the back of my arm didn't jiggle when I wave goodbye to my friends."

Kary's Story

I had spent many years as a teen and young woman not liking my body, then I grew to accept and love it as I became more immersed in fitness. I enjoyed the amazing changes my body went through as I grew stronger, leaner, and shapelier with weight training and proper nutrition. I even forgot about the ridicule I suffered from some of my junior high school peers about being "flat-chested." Then I started competing in women's fitness, the sport of the body beautiful!

In the beginning of my fitness career I was told that I would not do well in physique judging or fitness modelling if I did not get breast implants. This brought up a lot of uncertainty for me. I did not want to have any kind of unnecessary surgery, but the lure of looking good for the cameras and the fitness judges was strong. I started researching the subject of breast implants and even went in for a consultation with a surgeon.

Then I had the opportunity to listen to Michelle LeMay, a fitness celebrity and former sport aerobic competitor, speak at a fitness conference in Toronto. She spoke about the decisions people may make because of society's standards. Rarely do we see advertising depicting the inner qualities of people. Instead, we're bombarded with the superficial qualities, such as hair, body fat, facial beauty, breast size, etc. We all go through periods when we feel inadequate, and often we find ourselves comparing our physical attributes to those of others.

Many decisions about cosmetic surgeries are based on these comparisons and our ideas about what others want to see. Michelle referred to this as the voice of the ego. When you make a decision based on your ego, you are thinking about what the decision will mean to others. So before you make a decision, it is important to ask yourself how your true self really feels. Listen to your intuition or your inner voice—it always tells the truth. Base your decision on how you really feel and how it will affect your life, not on how others will react.

After hearing Michelle speak, I listened to my heart instead of my ego and I have never regretted my decision to remain au naturel. *The funny thing is, I did end up becoming a Pro Fitness competitor, I did end up competing with the best of the best, I did win Ms. Fitness Universe, and I did achieve my ultimate goal of qualifying for the Fitness Olympia contest. And I modelled in all the fitness magazines—flat-chest and all!*

Body-Image Boosters

I care not what others think of what I do, but I care very much about what I think of what I do. That is character!
—Theodore Roosevelt, 26th president of the United States

- Energy flows where attention goes, so focus on what you like most about yourself. Take charge of the degrading self-talk. Get out of the vicious cycle of attacking yourself with your thoughts. Focusing on parts you don't like can have negative effects on your entire outlook, which will spill over into your posture, words, and actions. Paying more attention to your good attributes (we're sure you can come up with at least one) will slowly make you feel better. Avoid body-bashing statements like, "My thighs are too big," and replace them with affirmations like, "I'm grateful to have strong legs that can move my body."

- Keep in mind the fact that people are attracted to others who are comfortable with their self-images. There are many telltale signs of a good body image: excellent posture, an easy smile, a confident stride, and maybe even a bounce to the step. These traits have universal appeal.

• Update your wardrobe or get a wardrobe makeover. Don't let yourself get stuck in an era. The '70s, '80s, and '90s were great decades, but those clothes should be long gone from your closet. Wear proper-fitting clothes that are clean and wrinkle-free; they enable you to exude comfort and confidence. Dress like you appreciate yourself right now instead of waiting for the ten pound weight loss.

• Do not participate in endless conversations about diet, food, and body weight. These discussions rarely end on a positive note. Have you ever noticed that you often leave those conversations feeling drained? Try and change the subject early in the conversation and don't feel the need to bash your own body in order to make others feel better.

• Acknowledge the fact that public opinion changes like the wind. In the Victorian Age, they admired plumpness. During the Roaring Twenties, thin was in. The '50s championed the hourglass figure. In the '60s, with the fascination of youth, culture, and freedom, models like Twiggy flourished. Do you want your body image to be dictated by public sentiment? Or do you want to be in the driver's seat of your own life?

• Start investing in the basics of good health and fitness, such as a good pair of walking shoes, a mountain bike, health-conscious cooking classes, supplements, or a subscription to informative magazines on lifestyle and wellness. Taking action is a great way to feel empowered.

• Motion drives emotion. It's hard to feel depressed when you are moving quickly and breathing deeply. Going for a walk gets the heart beating faster and blood circulating. The next level would be an aerobic workout or resistance training. The very act of exercising creates feel-good energy.

- Take care of yourself! Schedule massages or spend an entire day at a spa. Or create your own spa atmosphere at home with some scented candles and a hot bath. By spending time and energy on yourself, you are declaring that you are valuable!

- Be realistic! How much time and energy do you want to commit? A body with excellent muscle tone and low body fat (e.g., an Olympic gymnast or a ballerina) requires many hours of exercise per day and excellent eating habits. You can achieve a healthy level of fitness with a few hours invested per week. It is such a small amount of time when you consider that the average 65-year-old will have spent more than ten years of their life watching television.

- Stop comparing yourself with other people. We are all different shapes and sizes. At any given time, you will be either in better or worse condition than the people around you. Focus on how far you have come and celebrate each step you take from this day forward to add more peace of mind to your day.

Six Action Steps to Positive Thinking

The world is more malleable than you think, and it's waiting for you to hammer it into shape.
   —Bono, lead singer of U2

1. **For one day, be completely in tune with your thoughts**. Pay attention to everything you're thinking. Whenever an undesirable thought or picture enters your mind, substitute it with one that is pleasant. Think of your mind like a VCR—stop rewinding and replaying lousy scenes! Would you repeatedly watch a movie if you didn't enjoy it the first time?

2. **Have an arsenal of positive images for your personal, inner reference library**. Call this your positive emotional bank account. For example, recall:

- the time you achieved a personal best in an athletic event
- any special events or occasions with your family
- a job promotion or special task done well
- the completion of an important project
- the birth of a child
- a meaningful conversation with a mentor or loved one

3. **If you are feeling down, instead of reaching for coffee, the phone, or turning on the television, try some physical activity.** When you exercise, your blood gets pumping, and your respiration increases. In Chapter 6, "Goodbye Fat, Hello Fitness," we explain how exercise releases feel-good hormones called endorphins. One of our favorite phrases is "Motion creates emotion." When you feel good, you think better thoughts. It is the beginning of the miracle process.

4. **Make a list of positive self-affirmations and read them!** Carry them with you. It may sound corny, but we all need to be reminded of how special we are. In *You Can Heal Your Life*, Louise Hay reports that affirmations are a perfect way to reframe your negative self-talk. Louise has helped millions of people understand the power of affirmation. If, for example, you don't enjoy exercising and you keep saying, "I hate exercise," then it's very unlikely that you will ever develop a regular, consistent exercise habit. Oprah Winfrey has frequently stated: "I hate exercise," and we have all seen her ongoing challenge with her weight over the years. Our solution: Even though she may feel this way now, she has to stop declaring it publicly and privately. When her feelings of intense dislike start to bubble up, she could use a new health affirmation like: "This exercise is making me strong and giving me the energy to be a better role model for the people I inspire on a daily basis." Notice how we have linked her affirmation to one of her greatest values—helping others.

5. **Try listening to audiobooks while driving.** We often listen to audiobooks during long road trips. It's one of our favorite ways to spend less time on unproductive thinking. Visit your local bookstore and ask for the audiobook section. You can complete an audiobook in one week if you spend one hour per day in your car. That's fifty-

two books in one year. More books than most North Americans will read in a lifetime. Do you realize at this rate you will become an expert in any subject? Your car will be a university on wheels. We don't recommend listening to meditation tapes while you are on the road!

6. **Accept responsibility for all your words, deeds, and thoughts.** You can change your personal results only when you become accountable. Take notice any time you complain or lay blame. These victim attitudes decrease your personal power because you are affirming that something outside of yourself is responsible for your situation. You are telling yourself that you can't do anything about it. T. Harv Eker, in his *New York Times* best-selling book *Secrets of the Millionaire Mind*, reports that playing the role of a victim is a sure-fire way to guarantee that you will stay right where you are. Give yourself a mid-course correction. For example, you might say to yourself: "I am giving away my power right now." If you always blame your excess weight on frequent lunch meetings, you can take back your personal power by accepting responsibility and making healthier choices or scheduling meetings over tea instead!

Health Miracle Activities

1. Do you compare yourself to others or feel especially dissatisfied with yourself in certain situations?

_____

_____

2. What is your health mindset? What comes to mind when you hear the words "exercise" or "healthy eating"?

_____

_____

3. Is there a simple adjustment you could make in your self-talk as it pertains to your health mindset?

_____

_____

Chapter 3

The secret of getting ahead is getting started. The secret of getting started is breaking your complex, overwhelming tasks into small manageable tasks, and then starting on the first one.

—Mark Twain

Take Action—Today Not Tomorrow!

Even after years of abuse, if given the proper conditions, the body forgives the sins of the past and has the incredible capacity to heal itself, halt disease and revert to its rightful state of health and wellness.
　　—Dr. Joey Shulman

There is never a better time to *take action* than right now! Postponing forward momentum tells the universe that you are not ready for change, and certainly not ready to receive the benefits of the information you are acquiring by reading this book. Aim to do something within the first 24 hours of feeling inspired!

Psychologists have reported that when someone is ready for something new, it often makes an appearance. There is a reason why you picked up this book. We know you are ready for a new way of looking at health, wellness, and vitality. You are ready for a *health miracle*.

If you are reading this sentence at this moment, you are one of the people who are ready to enjoy the benefits of active living. We firmly believe that all things happen for a reason, and that more than just coincidence brought us together. We believe you have been looking for a solution to your health and fitness challenges. You know there is another way to feel in your body.

After speaking to thousands of people, we have concluded that one of the major keys to success is taking immediate action *today, not tomorrow!* That is how you ignite the fire within. Don't wait until Monday morning. And definitely don't put it off until January 1. Nothing will happen until you take action! The most successful people on the planet are action-oriented and we urge you to join them, starting with your health.

We had the opportunity to meet Mark Leblanc, 2008 president of the National Speaker's Association, while he was speaking to the Canadian Association of Professional Speakers (CAPS) in Toronto. He was lecturing on the topic of growing our speaking businesses. His main action step for his audiences was to commit to doing just one thing a day, five days per week, to get a new booking. He guaranteed that we would experience some amazing results. We were motivated! Only one thing a day, five days of the week? Surely this would be easy! We followed his advice and in the next month, we had booked four new speaking engagements! It was incredible! If only people would apply this concept to their health, just one action step per day, most days of the week. It is the stuff miracles are made of.

Seminar Attendee's Story

I [Kary] was recently approached before one of our seminars by a woman who did not look familiar to us. She embraced me and told me that I would probably not remember her, but she had come to the same seminar one year prior, hiding in the back row, overweight and downhearted about her life. She told me that she left our seminar with a strong feeling that she had to TAKE ACTION with one goal: stop drinking pop. She stopped drinking pop and six months later, she felt much better and had lost some weight. At that point she decided that if she could give up pop, she could do anything. So she made a few other changes to her diet and she started exercising. One year later, she stood before us, 50 pounds lighter and, in her own words, "with a whole new lease on life!"

Stop Postponing!

Think back to a time when you felt motivated after an inspiring song, movie, book, speaker, or conversation with a good friend, but something came up and your good intentions hit the backburner. You went about your regular routine. Days, weeks, and then months passed. And then you were another year older. Everyone has done it to some degree at one time or another. The spirit says yes, but the mind and body come up with excuses to wait!

When we postpone something we truly desire, the consequences are not obvious the first day or even the second. But days of postponing add up to another average year. A lifetime of average years will be filled with: "I wish I had . . ." "If only I'd . . ." "Why didn't I . . . ?" The years fly by quickly, and the excuses pile up, layer upon layer, brick by brick. The resulting wall imprisons you.

The Search for the Perfect Plan

If your ship doesn't come in, swim out to meet it.
  —Jonathan Winters, comedian

It sounds too easy. There must be some catch. Life is more complicated, right? Should I eat organic vegetables? Do I need to wash my vegetables with special detergent? Can they be frozen? How much should I eat? What about organic vegetables? Can I put special sauce or reduced-fat butter on them? Can I play first and eat after? Does it matter how hard I play or for how long? Can I play alone? The questions are endless, and by obsessively focusing on them, you indirectly postpone taking action. But the truth is *there is no perfect answer!*

Information about health and fitness is abundant, but information alone does not equal success! Some of you are waiting for that perfect article or health tip before you take the plunge. Let us break the news to you: If you continue to wait for something outside yourself, it may never come. You just need to move forward. It's often better to just get started than to try to figure it all out. Otherwise, you may end up wasting an entire life scratching your head, trying to figure out how to get things exactly right.

> ## *Health Miracle*
>
> **Heart disease is the #1 cause of death for American men and women. Studies show that exercising daily, not smoking, maintaining a healthy weight, and eating a nutritious diet can prevent more than 80 percent of heart disease. www.health.harvard.edu**

Feel the Fear and Do It Anyway!

If you listen to your fears you will literally die never knowing what a great person you might have been.
   —Robert Schuller, televangelist

Many people don't take action because they are afraid to fail. However, successful people know that failure is just one step on the ladder to the goal. It is part of the learning curve. Winston Churchill once said: "Success consists of going from failure to failure without loss of enthusiasm." Every failure comes with new information that you can apply to your next try, so celebrate the failures!

Over 30 publishers turned down the original manuscript for *Chicken Soup for the Soul*. That's 30 times the coauthors, Jack Canfield and Mark Victor Hansen, could have given up! They eventually found a publisher who was willing to take a chance, but they had to go into debt to prepurchase 20,000 copies for their own use and sales as part of the original contract. That first book sold 8 million copies and led to the series of 80 best-selling books.

Small Changes = Big Results

Simplicity is the key to brilliance.
   —Bruce Lee, martial arts legend

We recognize that changing your lifestyle is no easy task. Many of your habits have been with you since you were a toddler. Isaac Newton's first law of motion states that, "An object at rest tends to stay at rest and an object in motion tends to stay in motion unless acted upon by an outside force." No wonder it is so hard to get off the couch!

Think of the messages in this book as a prescription for reinvention. Let the stories and messages in *The Miracle of Health* be your force for change, the wind that fills the new set of your sail. You'll experience the benefits in all other areas. A ripple effect occurs when anyone takes charge of his or her health. The immediate benefit is a feeling of self-efficacy, and the next is an appearance of radiant energy. The sparkle in your eyes will tell the world you are alive and moving forward.

Laurie's Story

The day I stepped on my scale and saw 187 pounds was the day that I broke down and cried with the realization that I was going to end up like my recently deceased grandmother. Due to obesity, diabetes, and dementia-related complications, Grandma died in a nursing home, unable to care for herself or walk. In my mid-thirties, I was already experiencing poor health in the form of colitis. Luckily my sister and her husband are what you might call "health gurus," so I picked up my phone and took the first step. . . .

I asked Kary for a diet, but she refused. She told me that I needed to start making small, reasonable changes to my lifestyle that I could maintain forever. She reminded me that I needed to do this for the health of my children and husband, not just myself. I agreed to follow her suggestions and I started by recording my eating habits. It was obvious to my sister that major improvements were needed when she saw that I was drinking at least three or four colas per day. My sister explained to me that every can contains about 10 teaspoons of sugar, so I started having my cola treats on the weekend only! It was amazing—this was the only nutrition change we worked on for the first few weeks, plus I started working out at the gym in my office during my lunch break three or four times per week. I lost 10 pounds in the first month!

Slowly but surely, I changed over to whole grains, steamed veggies, fish, salads, fruits, and even some organic foods. I also started taking probiotics and omega-3 supplements. I incorporated weight training and cardiovascular training into my lunch-hour workouts every week, and tried to get the family out for walks and bike rides every weekend.

Fast-forward one year and I am a new woman! I have lost over 25 pounds of excess body fat and definitely feel stronger and more energetic than before. My whole family is benefiting from our new eating habits. Even my husband lost weight and we look forward to working out together as often as we can.

As for my health, I no longer need anti-inflammatory steroids like prednisone for my colitis. And my gastrointestinal specialist is amazed by my apparent control over my condition through eating and exercise. He actually wrote down the things I had changed so he could tell his other patients about them. He now refers to me as his "model patient."

Start with a Single Step

Take the first step in faith.
You don't have to see the whole staircase.
Just take the first step.
    —Martin Luther King Jr.

In the *Seven Spiritual Laws of Success*, Deepak Chopra said, "Within every seed is the promise of a thousand forests." A single seed falls on the ground, takes root, sends up a shoot, and becomes a tree. And then it, too, releases thousands of seeds in its lifetime.

You don't have to take 100 new health and fitness habits and make them yours. The attempt might seem noble, but the more you take on, the easier it is to fall off the wagon, and when that happens, it starts the cycle of self-doubt and self-loathing. Do what the title of best-selling author Judith Wright's book says and make *The One Decision*. This is the first step to success in any endeavor.

Health Miracle

You can raise healthy HDL cholesterol, lower bad LDL cholesterol, and decrease system-wide inflammation just by adding a few minutes of walking to every day.

Determination

Energy and persistence conquer all things.
    —Benjamin Franklin

Do you remember a specific time in your life when you put a massive amount of energy into getting something you really wanted? If you don't, then remember back to when you were a child and you wanted a special toy. Didn't you do whatever it took to get that toy? You bothered your parents daily, wrote letters to Santa, or prayed nightly. Remember leaving no stone unturned? The word "procrastination" wasn't in your vocabulary, and you did not believe in making excuses for not having the toy.

Can you imagine being able to harness that amount of determination and enthusiasm when you approach your health and fitness dreams as an adult? As you take that first step and begin to think about making a change in your life (which you are obviously doing right now!), then you must make a commitment and begin to act upon it *today!*

Think of children learning to take their first steps. Do they give up when they fall down? Of course not! What's more, everyone around them encourages them in their attempts. It may take months of trial and error, but most children eventually learn to walk. As the 13th President of the United States, Calvin Coolidge, once said, "Nothing in this world can take the place of persistence."

The Power of Choice

If you are not willing to risk the unusual, you will have to settle for the ordinary.
—Jim Rohn, author and business philosopher

The direction of our life's journey is carved by the choices we make. A single decision made in a pivotal moment can determine the quality of the following years. The decision postponed or never made will also affect your life. To doubt this is naive. To believe this is wisdom. To act on this is divine.

Most of us have the power to choose the quality and quantity of the food we put in our bodies. We also have the power to put down the TV remote and go for a walk. No one forces us to eat the next doughnut or skip our Monday afternoon workout. No one. It's the choices you continue to make every day that keep you looking and feeling the way you do.

Make It a Habit

Let us tell you a secret: Anyone can have better health and fitness if it's made a daily ritual. What do we mean by a ritual? Here's an example: Every day you probably do certain things at approximately the same time; you brush your teeth, eat, read, and go to work. These actions have become mindless because you have made them a part of your daily ritual. At first it takes effort to make something a daily ritual. We have to think about it and consciously do it. Yet in a surprisingly short amount of time (less than a month), it becomes a habit, changing our lives forever. (It has been said that it takes only 21 days to make a new activity a habit.)

Be prepared to feel a little anxiety or discomfort when you make those early changes in your lifestyle. The first steps in a new direction are always a little shaky and hesitant. Anyone who has decided to go in a different direction or break free from known boundaries has felt this, and that is where most people give up. They start to question themselves.

It is at those times that mental toughness and discipline must be in full force. Until you begin to feel and look better, the only thing that will keep you going in those early stages is your tenacity.

Health Miracle

Every minute 200 million new cells are renewed and re-energized in your body. The quality of the food you eat directly influences the developmental efficiency, revitalization, rejuvenation, and network communication functioning of each and every one of your cells.

—Sam Graci

Five Stages of Change

Our bodies are apt to be our autobiographies.
   —Frank Gillette Burgess, author and humorist

Have you heard the saying that the only ones who really enjoy a change are babies? Many people enjoy schedules, rituals, and predictable outcomes. "If it ain't broke, don't fix it" is a popular mantra. So, as health care advocates, we know that we are up against some tough odds when we promote a new way of life.

Change is one of the most powerful forces in nature. Just look to the seasons. Every spring washes away the dead of winter with new growth and promise. Summer follows and brings warmth and long days. With autumn comes the opportunity to harvest what you have sown. So goes the cycle of life.

Pyschologists Dr. James Prochaska and Dr. Carlo DiClemente wrote about the five stages of change. Recognizing which of the following stages you fit into can help you see what needs to happen before you can really enjoy and be comfortable with your experience. This is called the "maintenance" stage. When you finally arrive here, you no longer weigh yourself on a daily basis, count calories, and force yourself to exercise. Exercise and a healthy diet become part of your life.

1. **Precontemplation:** In this stage, you are not even thinking about healthy eating or exercising. You probably don't even recognize that what you eat has a huge impact on how you feel or how well your body functions. Exercise does not even cross your mind—you have "more important" things to worry about. If you are reading our book, we will assume that you are past this stage!

2. **Contemplation:** In this stage, you are just one decision away from taking action. A lot of people get stuck in this stage, getting ready to get ready. You might still be saying: "Some day I'll get started," and you recognize the fact that you probably should do something for your health. You notice information about health and you see family and friends either benefiting from good lifestyles or experiencing the negative consequences of poor health habits. You may have fleeting moments of imagining yourself taking some action. Leonardo da Vinci said, "Iron rusts from disuse; stagnant water loses its purity and in cold weather becomes frozen; even so does inaction sap the vigor of the mind."

3. **Preparation:** AHHHH . . . You are getting closer! You entertain the idea of joining a friend for a morning walk. You purchase a good pair of athletic shoes. You read the health advice column in your favorite magazine. You attend a health seminar. You come up with some fitness goals. You buy a book. You may have even brought up the issue of exercise and nutrition to your health care practitioner. You are poised and ready. . . .

4. **Taking action:** Finally! You have arrived! You lace up those sneakers and head out the door. You try one of the recipes from

your healthy living cookbook. You join your friend at the gym. You experience that first bead of sweat on your forehead and you proudly tell your friends and family about your newfound interests. **CAUTION:** This is a fragile stage and many people will never move beyond it. This is the stage where you easily fall off the wagon, have setbacks, and often get confused by the overwhelming amount of information that is available on health and wellness. Read to the end of the chapter for our five-pack action plan, which will help you stick to your new resolve.

5. **Maintenance:** Ralph Waldo Emerson said, "Do not believe that you can possibly escape the reward of your action." With persistence, determination, and some discipline come many benefits. Once healthy living has taken a firm footing, there is momentum in place. Eating nutritious food and making time for exercise becomes as effortless as brushing your teeth or driving your car. You know that exercise makes you feel good and you easily get back into your routine if you miss a day or two. You stop beating yourself up with guilt when you indulge in a piece of birthday cake and you no longer obsess about the amount of carbs in your dinner. You easily maintain your ideal weight and you finally accept and love your body.

Five-pack Action Plan

World-famous success coach Anthony Robbins, in his best-selling book *Awaken the Giant Within*, reported that all successful people leave clues behind them. Study these clues and you can learn how to achieve your own results. So, if you are interested in or, dare we say, committed to having high levels of results and fulfillment in your health and fitness endeavors, seek people who are achieving the kind of results you're looking for.

We have listed five clues that we have discovered in our search for people who are making it happen. Please note: Waiting around is not one of them!

1. **Decide:** Tell yourself that outstanding health and vitality are necessary in your life. Reaffirm on a daily basis that you are going to

take responsibility for the shape of your body. Successful people don't have an "I'll wait and see" attitude. They decide ahead of time that they will get the results they want.

2. **Schedule:** Sit down with your PDA, day planner, or calendar and make appointments for your fitness activities. Make it realistic and achievable. Even one exercise session per week for the rest of your life is better than starting out too vigorously and then quitting after three weeks of intense daily two-hour sessions. Studies have shown that doing a new activity at a scheduled time of day will help it become a permanent habit. When you reach the maintenance stage, you will be able to schedule your exercise with more flexibility because you will be less likely to talk yourself out of it!

3. **Share:** This strategy is about creating powerful alliances with your loved ones. You will be more likely to keep your commitment if your significant other or close friends are in it with you. This is a powerful tool and we go into more detail in Chapter 10, "Who Are You Flocking With?"

4. **Discipline:** Be strict with your new program. Getting close to your goals and then becoming lazy happens to most people who begin new healthy behaviors. They worked so hard to squeeze into the wedding dress or tux, and on the first day of the honeymoon, they fall right back into old habits. Carl Rowan said, "Nothing wilts faster than laurels that have been rested upon." Resting on your laurels starts slowly. You eat a little more one weekend. You miss your morning runs when work gets busy. Your sister from out of town visits for a week and she doesn't exercise. You conveniently neglect to weigh yourself all week and BAMM, you are five pounds heavier. People who are truly committed to lifelong health keep their nose to the grindstone, their finger on the pulse, their hands on the wheel. Yes, they do work harder at it, but they enjoy great rewards.

5. **Celebrate!** Reward yourself when you accomplish even the smallest goal. Don't wait until you have lost the entire 20 pounds before giving yourself permission to feel good. Get excited and reward yourself early, but not with food! Smaller goals that get rewarded in

the beginning give you a feeling of accomplishment and the sense that your goals are achievable. Every time you take a little step in the right direction, give yourself a pat on the back. Like a ripple effect, these initial steps will affect the other areas in your life.

Health Miracle

Most dieters postpone celebrating their achievements until the big weight loss. Research shows that even a 10-pound loss of unhealthy body fat can dramatically affect your bones, joints, sex organs, heart, and blood pressure in positive ways.

The Bottom Line

Don't wait. The time will never be just right.
　　—Napoleon Hill

You have to begin *now* to make those important health decisions. Yes, it is up to you. And yes, it's an inside job! You must start with the information you already know. Believe us, you know enough to get going. Take those first few steps on your own. These early steps are the beginnings of an incredible journey.

Rest assured that as you read *The Miracle of Health*, you will realize you deserve more than what you've been giving yourself and much more than what you've been settling for. No matter what kind of health and energy you and your loved ones currently have, there is a chance for you to make a change. Maybe this is your second, third, even twentieth chance. But it's your chance to make new decisions and take action. Life does not have to be the same again!

Health Miracle Activities

1. What current habits are taking you further away from how you want to look and feel?

　　＿＿＿＿＿＿＿＿＿＿＿＿＿＿＿＿＿＿＿＿＿＿＿＿＿＿

　　＿＿＿＿＿＿＿＿＿＿＿＿＿＿＿＿＿＿＿＿＿＿＿＿＿＿

2. Which of the five stages of change are you in?

_____

_____

3. What step could you take right now that will move you toward a healthier lifestyle?

_____

_____

4. Close your eyes and breathe deeply. See yourself taking action. See yourself taking that daily step toward how you want to look and feel. Picture how your life may change just by starting this one action step.

Chapter 4

Let food be your medicine and medicine be your food.
—Hippocrates

Conscious Eating

Health requires healthy food.
—Roger Williams, American theologian

The topic of eating is a hot one no matter how you slice it. The main purpose of food is to fuel the body, but for many, the relationship with food goes far beyond pure function. Family gatherings and celebrations are seen as a time to indulge. Time with friends is spent over lunch or dinner. Romantic evenings are long, drawn-out gustatory affairs. It seems like we are in a never-ending cycle of planning meals, preparing meals, serving meals, cleaning up after meals, or shopping for next week's meals. Throw in the discussions about where to go for dinner, and your life may seem like it revolves around food! Seeing food for what it really is—fuel for energy and growth—is one of the most important parts of gaining mastery over it.

Move a little more, eat a little less, breathe a little deeper, sleep a little longer, and make healthier choices. In a nutshell, this is the foundation for abundant health. Enough said. Thank you for reading this far. You can put the book down. You are on your own.

"Hey, wait a minute!" You are probably thinking, "There has to be more to it." You are right. If it's this easy, then why are more than half of Canadians and Americans overweight or obese and why are children *supersizing* themselves at an alarming rate? We are a well-educated society, aren't we? Yet, even health care professionals have problems with their weight.

You already know that you should be moving more and eating less—all the health books say that! So what are they not saying? What is the missing link to abundant energy and a healthy body?

Author and philosopher Sir Francis Bacon's famous quote, "Knowledge is power," doesn't seem to be true when it comes to health. We know we should eat well and move more. The challenge is putting your knowledge into action, enjoying the process, and maintaining your resolve. And going to the next level means helping a family member or friend. Being a role model and teaching the people you love healthy habits also strengthens your own daily disciplines. To be an authentic teacher, you must "walk the talk."

So what can we do to incorporate this knowledge into our lifestyle? That is the conundrum for most people. It is one thing to know better, and it is an entirely different thing to commit to doing better for life. And the jungle of "how to's" doesn't help. It's all so confusing. Just go online, type in "nutrition" and you will get over 169 million results. Try "fitness" and you will see more than 541 million. Type "diet" and you will get at least 212 million references. Good luck! There are too many choices and sources screaming for your attention. Unfortunately, information overload usually leads to paralysis by analysis. And we can't forget about those alluring promises and claims:

"Lose 30 pounds in 30 days!"
"Lose weight while eating cookies!"
"Lose 10 pounds in the first week!"

The list goes on and on.

Diet: A Nasty Four-letter Word

The second day of a diet is always easier than the first. By the second day, you're off it.
—Jackie Gleason, comedian

When someone loses weight, it seems like everyone within 10 miles wants to know how he or she did it! "What diet are you on?" "What did you take?" are the first questions that pop up. Author Dan Bennett said,

"Probably nothing in the world arouses more false hopes than the first four hours of a diet."

One in four men and one in three women are on a diet at any one time in North America. If diets worked, the $30 billion a year spent on the diet industry would be making a dent in the number of overweight people. Yet the truth is statistics show otherwise: the obesity problem is getting worse and 95 percent of all dieters regain lost weight within two years!

Obsessively controlling food adds a false sense of structure and certainty to a day. Chronic dieters get the opportunity to feel special every time they explain their new eating regimens. When the quick fix ends with failure, the dieter often receives consolation and connection with others who have also "fallen off the wagon." This becomes a seductive, but never-ending cycle.

There's nothing mysterious or magical about decreasing your body weight on any diet. The Zone, The Blood Type Diet, Atkins, South Beach, Pritikin, Sugar Busters, The Cabbage Soup Diet, The Apple Diet, The Maple Syrup Diet, and The Scarsdale Diet all promote restriction of calories. Of course you will initially lose some weight if you can follow the stringent rules of any diet, but can you actually maintain the results over a lifetime?

A fad diet will rarely give you permanent, healthy results. For most, the diet will keep the weight off only as long as you're on that particular diet. The moment you leave the caloric restriction of the diet, the weight creeps (or somersaults) back on. Most end up with more body fat than they originally had because of the slower metabolism, lost muscle tissue, and binge-like behavior that usually follows a diet. But if you change your habits—your lifestyle—you *can* make a permanent change. And you can still enjoy some indulgences without guilt!

Jill's Story

I'm a walking nutritional database. I have tried every diet on the market. I can tell you about fat grams, calories, glycemic index—you name it. I'm heavier now than when I first started riding the diet roller-coaster. And I'm preoccupied with the enemy—food.

I go out for dinner with friends or family and put up a brave front. I pick at a plain, lifeless salad and eat very little. Later on, I eat alone

(continued)

in the comfort of my home, where I can eat whatever I want. I feel stuck. I cannot bear the thought of going on another diet, but I need to lose this weight.

Dean and Sandy's Story

We once asked a nutritionist how many calories we would have to burn or not eat in order to lose about 2 pounds per week. She explained that every 2 pounds would require a caloric deficit of about 1,000 calories per day or 7,000 calories per week. We did the math and realized that we would have to give up a lot of food and exercise for more than 90 minutes every day to achieve this. Our nutritionist asked if this was a reasonable expectation for our busy lives. We knew that it would be impossible to maintain for more than a few weeks.

Our nutritionist then explained that by cutting only 100 calories per day (the equivalent of a medium-size cookie or a small soft drink) and aiming for 30 minutes of physical activity most days of the week, we could achieve fat-loss results over the course of the year that would benefit our health and would be maintainable. The best part was that we would not be changing our current lifestyle drastically. She also explained that over time, as we felt better, we would probably be encouraged to adopt more healthy habits, which would increase our chances of even more fat loss over the long term.

One year later we are both more than 10 pounds lighter and our zest for life has increased exponentially. Our medical doctors have applauded our efforts and were excited to see an improvement in our health profiles and blood pressure. It wasn't that hard to stop eating one cookie every day and we really look forward to our evening walk. We also started eating a large salad with protein as one of our meals most days of the week. This year we have a goal to start resistance training two times per week and we are looking to make a few more changes to our diet. We may even sign up for a weekly dance lesson. Our nutritionist says that we can expect at least another 10-pound weight loss with our new goals. The best part is that neither of us feels restricted and we know that these changes are permanent!

Are Your Eyes Bigger than Your Stomach?

My doctor told me to stop having intimate dinners for four. Unless there are three other people.
— Orsen Welles, Academy Award–winning director

Overeating is a fairly common phenomenon. If you look back some 100,000 years (long before the drive-thru restaurant), there was no government to regulate production and storage of food. Refrigeration did not exist, so in times of excess, people engaged in frenzied eating to celebrate. And in times of famine, extra body fat was an asset.

> **Did You Know?**
> *Dieting by itself without exercise leads to a slower metabolism and lost lean body mass or muscle tissue, the tissue that gives you the strength to complete daily tasks.*

In the Western world, we have such a challenging time pushing ourselves away from the table or the fridge. It's hard to stop in the moment because it tastes *sooo* good as it goes "down the hatch." But you pay the price minutes later when you struggle to get out of your chair! There are health consequences to overeating. Your entire digestive system must work overtime as it takes a massive amount of energy to break down a large volume of food into its usable components. This leaves you with less energy for the other important areas in your life—your family, your career, your friends, and your hobbies.

The stomach is a very flexible organ. Overeating stretches the stomach beyond its natural size. It will not return to its natural size if it is constantly (at every meal) being stretched beyond its limits. This larger stomach will require more and more food to satisfy your perceived hunger. When you begin to eat with sound nutritional principles, it will take a while before that stretched stomach starts to regain its natural dimensions. That is why the first few weeks of nutritious eating may seem very challenging. We guarantee that over time, your body will get used to the new amounts of food, and you will feel satisfied with smaller portions.

The urge to overeat is so powerful, it is no wonder we are the fattest people on the planet. At the rate we are expanding our waistlines, researchers like Dr. Beverly White, Ph.D., R.D., and Dr. Barbara Brehm from Smith College estimate that by 2030, over 90 percent of the population will be overweight. Frightening! Isn't this enough to make you want an apple instead of a brownie?

Did You Know?

There are currently 1.3 billion people on the planet suffering from diseases related to overeating and inactivity. At the same time, about 1 billion people are suffering from the ill effects of malnutrition.

Are you constantly tired or wonder why you don't have the energy you ought to? Do you rely on coffee or other caffeinated drinks to get through the day? Is your concentration lacking at certain times of the day? Do you experience heartburn, indigestion, bloating, fatigue, mood swings, or flatulence? Or have long-term consequences of a poor diet and overeating become your daily battle: obesity, diabetes, heart disease, loss of mobility, joint problems, poor self-image, eating disorders, social isolation, depression, or even cancer?

Most people are aware that their food consumption has an effect on how they feel, yet they regularly overeat. They justify their behavior by saying, "I missed breakfast," "It's a special occasion," "It's free," "My eyes were bigger than my stomach," or "I can't let it go to waste; there are people starving in some parts of the world."

Obviously this is an area that needs to be addressed! Unless the underlying reasons are identified, you may always find yourself unbuckling your belt at the dinner table.

Food Cravings and Addictions

A happy mind automatically thinks happy thoughts, and a healthy body automatically hungers for healthful foods.
  —John Gray, author and psychologist

Food is such an emotional topic. Just question any mother on how she feeds her children if you like a heated debate! Or ask people about their memories of family gatherings: their eyes will glaze over and get a little misty when they mention Mom's apple pie, Grandma's chocolate chip cookies, or the breakfast Dad made on Sundays. With that much emotion tied into the subject, it's no wonder a huge wall of resistance comes up with the mention of a change in diet.

We eat when we're hungry, but we also tend to eat when we're stressed, bored, unhappy, anxious, or lonely. Perhaps we eat to temporarily take our minds off our woes. With a pail of ice cream and soup spoon in hand, we get completely absorbed in the physical moment. Breathing deepens, colors brighten, and a feeling of euphoria fills us. Memories of happier times and feelings often flood back. Feel-good hormones saturate our brains. And we link all these feelings to the *food*.

It doesn't take a degree in psychology to see that food helps us cope. Who hasn't gone to the fridge for some ice cream when they're down in the dumps? It very easily becomes a habit to head for the kitchen whenever we feel things are not going well. And why does it seem like the foods we crave are always the ones that are high in sugar and/or fat? How often have you reached for a salad when you're feeling blue? Elizabeth Somer, R.D., wrote about this connection in *Food & Mood*. She emphasized that it's only a temporary fix and, if done often enough, it can lead to unwanted weight gain.

Health Miracle

The movement toward a life of health and vitality can begin with a simple shift in your thinking. Joe Dispenza said, "Every single cell in your body is spying on your thoughts." Positive thoughts provide a supportive environment for optimal functioning; negative thoughts undermine your wishes for health and vitality.

How to Conquer Your Food Cravings

Everyone makes about 250 food decisions a day. . . . Should I have coffee? Should I put milk in it? Whole or skim? Sugar, Splenda, Stevia?
—Professor Brian Wansink

Sleep: In his book, *Sleep 101*, Steve Stone reported that half of American adults experience sleep difficulties. It's a 24/7 world. Students e-mail their teachers at 3 a.m., and an abundance of channels on the television give you a nonstop diet of news and entertainment. With so many distractions pulling people away from their beds, people are losing sleep. Back in 1910 people used to sleep an average of nine hours a night. In 2008, Dr. Norman Shealy reported that the average American sleeps about five to six hours per night. Reduced pillow time means that your body has less chance to rejuvenate and replenish from your day's activities. Important hormones like growth hormone (needed for growth and reproduction), melatonin (needed for deep sleep, proper immune function and sexual appetite), and serotonin (needed for regulation of emotions and metabolism) are adversely affected. Long-term sleep deprivation leads to higher levels of the stress hormone cortisol in your system and stronger cravings for all things sweet. The end result: unwanted pounds. In a long-term study of 68,000 middle-aged women, researchers from Case Western Reserve University in Cleveland found that those who slept five hours or less per night were 32 percent more likely to be overweight than those who slept seven hours.

Decrease stress: Are you desperately seeking balance? Unmanaged stress will also make you fat. If you are unable to keep an even keel, you will be more likely to have spikes of the hormone cortisol. Elevated levels of this hormone lead to increased heart rate, shallow breathing, and the disruption of digestion. It's ironic that when cortisol levels increase, you want to eat. The very foods you are driven to eat will not be digested properly. The resulting bloating, stomach upset, and flatulence will have you running to the drug store. When you have a craving try deep breathing and other relaxation techniques. Len Krawitz, Ph.D., has shown that by taking some deep diaphragmatic breaths, you can change your physiological state from one of anxiety to one of calm. While your mind is quiet, you can ask yourself if you are truly hungry or simply experiencing an emotional response and looking for distraction. See Chapter 11, "Desperately Seeking Balance" for more on stress and relaxation.

Balance your meals: At most meals, aim to eat carbohydrates (like brown rice, whole-grain products, and starchy vegetables) with protein (for example, chicken, fish, lean red meat, and eggs). Registered dieticians report that eating a balanced meal gives your body more sustained energy. When your body is getting what it needs at mealtime, you decrease the likelihood of grabbing a quick-fix snack. The average chocolate bar has more than 250 calories—even 120 extra calories a day beyond your normal requirements will lead to a 1-pound weight gain per month! Doesn't seem like much the first month, but at the end of the year, you will need to purchase some larger clothes.

Exercise: Does this recommendation surprise you? Movement will raise levels of your body's own feel-good chemicals, helping you to decrease stress and anxiety. It also increases your lung efficiency and cardiac output, builds muscle, burns calories, and makes you more flexible. Exercise can make you look great and feel good, and it's hard to wolf down potato chips when you're on the treadmill!

Music: It can change the way you feel and energize you if you're bored or relax you if you're stressed. Music has the marvelous ability to change your state of mind. Most people do not binge eat when they feel good, so blast out some of your favorite tunes! Some of our favorite artists are: Enya, Mozart, Vivaldi, and Andrea Bocelli.

Call a friend: A good conversation with a friend can help distract you from any craving—unless they're working at a take-out restaurant. Peace Pilgrim once said, "Make food a very incidental part of your life by filling your life so full of meaningful things that you'll hardly have time to think about food."

Make a deal: A pact or fun contract with your significant other or best friend could inspire you to new disciplinary heights. Maybe you will make a deal to brew your own coffee at home instead of stopping at the local coffee shop where you frequently indulge in high-calorie beverages and sweet treats.

Drink water: You would be surprised how often people mistake dehydration for hunger. See the next chapter, "The Miracle of Health: Nutritional Recommendations," for more information about water and its astounding effects on the human body.

Just say no! Develop your mental gymnastics. If a torte or a honey-glazed doughnut tempts you, remember your decision to choose healthier food. Ask yourself if a poor choice will work against your new health and fitness goals. Just saying *no* strengthens self-discipline. It feels good to walk away from a dessert or a high-calorie treat. You can walk a little taller knowing you're better than the doughnut. Okay, we're getting a little silly. But the point is to say *no* to debauchery and *yes* to sound nutrition. American artist and writer Florence Scovel Shinn said, "Nothing on earth can resist an absolutely non-resistant person." Basically, a strong resolve creates an inner calm that unsupportive outside forces are unable to penetrate.

Cognitive restructuring: This is a type of therapy that brings awareness to a person's thought processes. If you have intense food cravings that aren't serving you, cognitive therapy might be an excellent way to develop a healthy attitude toward food. Author and speaker Les Brown says, "What you resist will persist." In other words, you may end up thinking about the *demon doughnuts* all day if you never address the underlying emotional issues. Dr. Deepak Chopra says that simple awareness of the personal challenge at hand can initiate healing. Take the time to ask yourself what you are really feeling before you grab the food. There's no shame in counselling if that's what it takes to break out of the prison of destructive feelings and behaviors.

Mindful Eating

Of course we have free will. Free will resides in our frontal cortex [lobe], and we can train ourselves to make more intelligent choices and to be conscious of the choices we're making.
    —Candace Pert, Ph.D

Mindful eating is your personal solution to the barrage of advertising to *eat* and *eat* and *eat* some *more*. Nurturing your mind to think consciously about food will give you an armor of protection to combat every tactic marketers use to get you in the store and buy their products. The rest of this chapter is devoted to making you a more mindful eater.

Uche's Story

I have never met anyone who has eaten at McDonalds more times in a day than I have. Can you guess how many? Well, it was three times in a single day! It was many years ago when I first started practising dentistry. And it was on a day that I worked 12 hours. I went through the drive-thru at noon, then again on my dinner break. On the way home later that evening, I felt I deserved a "break today" and went through and ordered a Big Mac, shake, and fries for the third time. By midnight I had special sauce oozing out of parts of me you wouldn't believe. I tossed and turned all night and couldn't believe I had spent $20 to feel that badly!

The Magic of Journalizing

Always bear in mind that your own resolution to succeed is more important than any other one thing.
—Abraham Lincoln, 16th president of the United States

In the beginning, you need to keep track to get on track. Record where you were, when and what you ate, and how you felt before and after the food. After a few days you will have a greater awareness of your bad habits and triggers for poor choices. You will be more mindful. A health care professional will be able to easily identify vitamin and mineral deficiencies and make recommendations if you can provide written records of what you normally eat.

Most people think they are doing okay when asked about their eating habits. You may be surprised at the reality of yours. People routinely underestimate how many empty calories they eat

Did You Know?
A large study funded by the U.S. National Heart, Lung, and Blood Institute compared the fast-food habits of young adults over a period of 15 years. One group ate at these venues more than twice per week and the other group less than once per week. At the end of the study, the participants who frequented fast-food restaurants more than twice each week had gained an extra 10 pounds, and had a significant increase in insulin resistance, which is a risk factor for type 2 diabetes.

and overestimate how many nutrient-rich foods are in their diets. Nobel Prize–winner Al Gore, in his award-winning documentary *An Inconvenient Truth*, quoted Mark Twain: "It ain't what you *don't know* that gets you into trouble. It's what *you know for sure* that just ain't so."

Health Miracle

The American Psychological Association concurs that recording food intake will help create awareness of eating behaviors. Patients report that it is one of the best obesity-management tools and research has consistently shown that it improves treatment outcomes.

Slow Down!

Have you ever found yourself wolfing down a meal while talking on the phone, or driving the car, or preparing for a family outing? When you eat quickly, your food rarely gets broken down properly. Your stomach doesn't have teeth! Large chunks in your stomach require the acids to work overtime to finish the breakdown process. Digestive problems of all kinds can result.

Can you guess where digestion starts? No, it's not in the mouth. It's with your nose and eyes. You first smell the roast cooking. You see the juices glistening through the oven window. You mouth salivates and your stomach releases enzymes in preparation for the upcoming meal. Racing through a drive-thru and gobbling down the food in the car leaves little time for seeing, smelling, and savoring a meal.

Eat slowly in a relaxed atmosphere and avoid other activities while eating. Make an effort to chew thoroughly and enjoy the taste of your food. You will get more satisfaction and better nutritional value if you eat this way. Try to eat at the table instead of while watching television or while standing at the counter reading the mail or returning your phone calls. Jonathan Goldman, author of *Healing Sounds*, suggests listening to slow music while you dine.

Health Miracle

It takes about 20 minutes for the stomach to signal the brain that it's full. Just by slowing down your meals, you can avoid overeating, so your brain will actually have the time to signal that you are full. Try putting your fork down between bites!

Who Needs Breakfast?

When you skip meals, you deny yourself the regular intake of fuel and nutrients you require to function efficiently. Meal skippers tend to experience many energy highs and lows in their days. They may actually feel light-headed or irritable after not eating for many hours.

Skipping breakfast can lead to unhealthy choices later in the morning. Research has shown meal skippers are more likely to be overweight because they overeat later in the day to compensate for the missed meals. Meal skippers often have poor eating habits, which, combined with stress, can leave them vulnerable to illness.

Eating a healthy breakfast bumps up your metabolism in the morning and helps complete the digestive process from the day before. Preparing and eating a morning meal can be a challenging habit to develop, but the payoff is worth it. You can start with just a piece of fruit and some nuts or one of those delicious meal-replacement bars or smoothies. Our favorites can be found in Chapter 5.

Are you still thinking, "Who needs breakfast? I get my early morning kick from coffee." Did you know that coffee gives you a false energy boost and can be addictive and dehydrating? Seventy percent of soft drinks also contain caffeine. Beware! Being a caffeine junkie can lead to headaches, anxiety, and insomnia. So, avoid using coffee to replace a meal, and enjoy it in moderation.

Health Miracle

Studies on individuals who have maintained long-term weight loss show that they regularly eat breakfast.

Portion Control

If you eat too much today, you choose to weigh too much tomorrow.
    —Uche Odiatu

Many of us are confused about how much food we should eat at each meal. The U.S.D.A. Food Pyramid and the Canada Food Guide recommend specific portion and serving sizes. For example, a serving of vegetables or starchy carbohydrate (brown rice or pasta) is the amount you could fit in half a regular coffee cup. A serving of salad would be a full cup. A serving of meat would be the size of a deck of cards. Beware: In this age of huge portions, it's possible to eat all your daily recommended calories at one sitting.

> **Resource:**
> **www.nhlbi.hih.gov**
> *Search "portion distortion quiz" for a fun look at how portions have changed and how much exercise you need to do to burn off the extra calories.*

Start with baby steps. If you regularly ask for seconds, you might limit yourself to only one plate—maybe you need a smaller plate! After a few weeks, you will get used to your new habit. Remember to eat slowly, so you can stop eating before you are bursting at the seams. Perseverance will pay off, and you will eventually find that you require less food to fill up.

Eat Lightly at Night

Did you know your body requires more fuel during the first half of the day than it does as it winds down for the evening? "Eat breakfast like a king; eat lunch like a lord; and supper like a pauper." What happens when you do the reverse? Well, people who tend to eat more during the second half of the day are more prone to storing the food as body fat. Brad King, author of *Fat Wars*, reported that optimal fat-burning can occur if you go to bed on an empty stomach. This best-selling author goes on to say that this habit will slow the aging process and lead to optimal health.

A large meal should end about three hours before you go to bed. A lighter meal could take place up to two hours before bedtime and a small, nutritious snack could be eaten one hour before sleep. This gives your body a chance to digest most of the food before you go to sleep. After eating, your insulin levels rise and prevent melatonin from spiking. Melatonin enables you to sleep deeply. According to researcher Sam Graci, melatonin is also your system-wide, natural anticancer hormone. Over many years, eating large meals late at night will severely diminish melatonin levels.

Most of the repair work in the body is done during the latter part of the evening and overnight. While you are sleeping, your body attempts to rejuvenate and detoxify every organ. Yes, ladies, this includes your skin! If your body is too busy digesting food while you sleep, not only will you wake up feeling tired, you will accelerate the aging process of every organ in your body, so go to bed with your significant other, not a croissant!

Out of Sight, Out of Mind

Eliminate any food in your house that has not been chosen with sound nutritional principles. Now you'll avoid the midnight rendezvous with your refrigerator. You may be thinking: "What about the kids?" or "We need to have treats for our guests." But remember: if the average person ate two fewer cookies each day at 60 calories each with no other nutrition or exercise changes, he or she would lose around 10 pounds in a year.

High-sugar treats are very addictive. Sure, they are comfort foods, but if eaten to excess, you will be dealing with an increasing waistline, large thighs, and a double chin.

Sugar has been found to trigger the release of opiates (feel-good chemicals) in the brain. This high is short-lived and is followed by a crash in energy every time. This is a physiological fact. You hear people say, "Oh, I need some quick-energy food." But what they fail to realize is that the quick high is followed by an insulin spike—your body thinks it is an emergency and socks it away in your liver and muscles. Low blood sugar follows, which leads to a rise in cortisol and adrenalin. Like cortisol, adrenalin is a fight-or-flight brain messenger. They both warn your body of an emergency and cause a series of physiological responses: the heart rate speeds up, breathing becomes rapid, your blood clots easier, and digestion slows. As soon as you experience the low blood sugar, you start looking for your next pick-me-up. It is a destructive, vicious cycle that is played out daily for many of the overweight people in North America

So get rid of the unhealthy treats that are stockpiled in most households. Who hasn't finished an entire bag of potato chips during a TV movie and then exclaimed, "I can't believe I ate all of that!" Having no junk food in your house might sound extreme, but the results are amazing! The best part is you can actually enjoy the dessert at the restaurant or party if you regularly eat with sound nutrition principles at home.

Eating Out, Not Pigging Out!

Challenge
Put down this book right now and take an inventory of your kitchen. Take everything that is considered "junk food," and put it into a box and get rid of it. This will definitely be a challenge if you have been raised in a family with constant reminders of "All the starving people in the world . . ."

Dining out at restaurants is an unavoidable part of today's world. John Naisbitt, in his best-seller *Megatrends 2000*, reported that 40 cents of every food dollar is spent in restaurants. And we are not talking about fine dining: it's happening at fast food restaurants. The following is a list of suggestions that will help you face your next restaurant dining experience with anticipation rather than apprehension.

1. Before you leave for the restaurant, commit yourself to making healthier food choices. Cathy Jameson, Ph.D., says "The first step to success is deciding to be a success." Decide ahead of time that you will stick to the healthier choices on the menu. Many restaurants offer these options, so don't be afraid to ask the waiter for recommendations. You don't even have to open the menu, and you could even enjoy a slice of bread! Ask for plain bread and dip it in olive oil and balsamic vinegar instead of coating it with artery-clogging butter.

2. Don't starve yourself all day if you are heading out to eat. It is a mistake to believe that skipping meals throughout the day gives you an excuse for overeating when you go out. Your body can utilize only so many calories at one meal and the rest will be stored as body fat. And starving yourself makes your metabolism slow down, which is counterproductive to becoming a *fat-burning* machine.

3. Don't read the menu like it's a letter from your lover! Menus are designed to tantalize and entice you into overeating. Of course you can enjoy the dining-out experience, but try to put more focus on your company, the conversation, and the ambiance.

4. Order with conviction. You set yourself up for failure the minute you waiver in your intention and start asking what other people are going to order. It might sound like you are being personable, but people admire someone who can make a quick decision. Certainty is very attractive! Take the lead and set the tone for a healthy, life-giving meal. If you have children with you, remember that they learn by watching. Set them up for a lifetime of healthy eating.

5. Ask for dressings and sauces (which contain many artery-clogging fats) on the side, so you have control over the quantity you consume. Most restaurants have lighter choices or, even better, an olive oil and vinegar mix.

6. Order an entrée only. If you must have a dessert or appetizer, share! There are some very easy ways to cut back on the total calories in your dining-out experience. Eating a broth-based soup (not cream) before a meal usually means that 25 percent less food gets eaten. Isn't that interesting? Think how many calories you'd avoid if you did that every time you ate out.

7. If you are having a dense meal (meat, starchy carbohydrates, and vegetables), say *no* to the breadbasket. We know it's free—and who doesn't like free stuff—but it adds to your total meal calorie count.

8. As the day goes on, your need for large, high-calorie meals diminishes. So, if you are out for a late dinner, stick to choices made from vegetables, salads, and lower-fat protein sources (e.g., fish,

chicken, or extra-lean cuts of red meat). Research has shown that overweight people are inclined to consume more meals later in the day compared to people of average weight.

9. Always aim to leave some food on your plate. We know it is a small act, but this demonstration of discipline will help you feel like you have power over your eating habits. This sends a very clear message to yourself and to the universe that you are serious.

10. Enjoy your company more than the food! Think of dining out as a vehicle to strengthen relationships. Focusing on the conversation and your dining companions will also enable you to eat slower.

Shopping Strategies

You've got bad eating habits if you use a grocery cart in a 7-Eleven.
    —Dennis Miller, comedian

It is much easier to stay on track with your resolve if you attempt to integrate healthy living principles into every part of your day. Bill Phillips in *Eating for Life* said, "Eventually, anyone and everyone who's at all concerned with their health must learn how to feed their body, not starve it." If you make good food choices at the supermarket, you know you have given yourself a head start.

✓ **Begin with the end in mind.** Stephen Covey's *Seven Habits of Highly Effective People* is not just for business success. Keep your health and fitness goals in mind while you prepare a list of excellent food choices. Having clear intentions can streamline your fitness journey. Deepak Chopra, in *The Seven Spiritual Laws of Success*, discusses how focused intentions and desires can enhance any experience. Look at shopping as a means of getting the fuel for your life's journey.

✓ **Eat before you go.** Will you be strong in your intention if your stomach is growling and begging for attention? Food choices are markedly different with hunger nipping at your heels. That bag of cheese-flavored tacos and Oreos that you bought for future company will not make it past the "front-seat feeding frenzy" if you are famished.

✓ **Avoid shopping at the end of a long, stressful day.** It's very easy to justify poor choices if you are tired and in a hurry to get home. Checking labels and reaffirming your sound nutrition mission statement will be the furthest thing from your mind! Coaching legend Vince Lombardi said, "Fatigue makes cowards of us all."

✓ **Stick to the perimeters of the supermarket.** It is not an accident that most of the healthiest food choices (fish, poultry, lean meats, fruits, veggies, eggs, and soy milk, for example) are tucked away on the outskirts of the store, requiring a walk through the other aisles. By the time you reach the fruit and vegetables you will have been tempted to purchase a bag of chips and a box of cookies.

✓ **Fresh is best.** Canned foods have lost some of their nutrient content due to the high heat and pressure they are subjected to in the canning process. These items are usually higher in salt as well. There are a number of studies reporting that canned foods may expose people to potentially harmful levels of Bisphenol A or BPA—an estrogen mimicker. BPA has been linked to disruption of vital organs.

✓ **Live foods are an essential part of a nutritious diet.** When choosing fresh fruits and vegetables, look for brightly colored items with little or no bruising or marking. Check for firmness, and do not hesitate to ask when the next shipment of fresh produce is expected. Most stores have a specified day of the week when they receive their produce. It's smart to shop within the next day or two, so you get the best quality and variety.

✓ **Be careful at the checkout counter.** These areas are geared for impulse buying. There has been much research on buying habits. Store owners then use this knowledge when they set up the counters with their inviting displays of candies and other treats.

✓ **Beware of the fat-free foods.** Fat free does not mean calorie free. It is easy to be misled into thinking that fat-free foods are healthy. A lot of fat-free foods contain about the same amount of calories as their regular counterparts. Many of them contain even more processed chemical components and are high in sugar.

✓ **Read labels.** Checking food labels is a great habit. Taking the time to read them means you're taking responsibility for what goes into your body. By examining the labels, you will see the chemical additives, preservatives, salt, sugar, and fat content of what you're eating. It is an enlightening experience when you find out what you are putting into your body. The statement, *you are what you eat,* takes on an entirely new meaning. Studies have shown that people who read the labels on food packages are more likely to make healthier food choices. Here are a few common words used on food packaging:

- *Low Fat:* A product that has 3 grams or less of fat per serving. (Remember, there may be more than one serving in a package!)
- *No added sugar:* This does not necessarily mean sugar-free. It simply means it is processed without additional sugar.
- *Lite:* Items that contain one-third less calories than the original item. (Not necessarily low fat.)

By simply being aware of the ingredients in your food, you'll make better choices. You'll begin to ask yourself the question: "Will this food item take me closer to the way I want to look and feel or further away?" This question can make the entire shopping experience much easier and more interesting. Making more conscious food choices will take your gustatory experience to a new level. *New York Times* best-selling author Eckhart Tolle in his book *A New Earth* reports that anytime you become more conscious during your day, your life will take on new meaning.

✓ **Try something new.** Don't bury your head in the sand: Ostrich meat has less fat than commercially raised lamb, beef, chicken, turkey, or pork. It also has fewer calories, less cholesterol, and the same amount of protein per serving. It costs more per pound than beef, but the fact that it has no bones or fat makes the price worth it. Did you know ostrich cooks in half the time compared to beef and does not shrink unless overcooked?

✓ **Don't hesitate to tell your grocery managers that you are interested in organic and free-range foods.** They will be more likely to stock these items if they know that consumers are looking for them. Just think, you are not only taking charge of your own health, but you are helping others as well.

80/20 Rule

All personal breakthroughs begin with a change in beliefs.
  —Anthony Robbins, author and motivational speaker

At each mealtime, ask yourself if the food you are about to eat will help or hinder you in your quest for better health. Another recommendation is to eat well 80 percent of the time with "food for function" in mind. This will allow for those special occasions and times when it is almost impossible to say no, like on your birthday!

Give up that all-or-nothing attitude! We often hear people say that once they have eaten one cookie, they may as well finish the entire row. This all-or-nothing mindset often leads to a whole day of bingeing. Having one cookie does not mean you have "blown" your decision to eat healthily. Do not write off a day because you overate at one meal! Reaffirm your healthy intentions, and move forward. *Remember, strive for excellence, not perfection!*

Robert's Story

I was sick and tired of the way I looked and felt. I tried to do everything at once. I gave up my coffee, I threw out my cookies, and I vowed to never eat chocolate again! Bye-bye banana splits. I hired a trainer and saw a registered dietitian. I purchased a membership at my local gym and a treadmill for my 6:00 a.m. cardio workout.

For the first week, I managed to exercise two hours per day and did not veer from my established eating plan. During the second week, I began wondering when the miraculous transformation would take place. How come I still looked the same?

My family was feeling alienated by my Navy Seals training regimen—even the dog was avoiding me. By the end of the second week, I found myself in a drive-thru wolfing down a double burger, fries, and a shake.

Health Miracle

Eating dark chocolate can decrease blood pressure as effectively as some of the most common hypertensive medications according to recent studies. It can also lower LDL (lousy) cholesterol and boost HDL (good) cholesterol.

Stay On the Path

Good food will nourish us without causing stress, and thus allow our immune system to spend its energy in healing.
—Annemarie Colbin

Relapse is normal, and it is important to acknowledge this. By accepting the facts, you can prepare yourself for a momentary slip or poor judgment. Instead of feeling guilty and falling completely off the wagon, you can simply admit that you slipped up and then use some of the following strategies to move ahead with your goals:

- Identify high-risk situations like weddings, birthday parties, etc., and make an action plan before you leave the house. Maybe you will sit with someone who eats healthy foods, or maybe you will eat a small meal before the event so that you will not be overly hungry when you arrive. Try a meal-replacement bar or a piece of fruit with some unsalted nuts. You can also drink a couple of glasses of water before you leave for the event.

- Have a coping response. You might remind yourself of your health goals and powerful reasons. Or maybe you have a mantra that you can repeat to yourself: "Will this next choice take me closer toward or further away from how I want to look and feel?" Or "I am a lean, toned, athletic machine."

- Visualize yourself making good decisions and healthy choices and see yourself saying *no* to overindulgence. Solomon in Proverbs 29:18 said, "Without a vision, the people will perish." Hey, take it one step further: "With a vision you will flourish."

- If you do slip up, forgive yourself and view it as a learning experience. Ask yourself what you learned and what you could do better next time. No one becomes overweight in a single meal. It is the habit of consistently overeating and making poor food choices that creates a distorted body shape.

- Find tasty recipes for good health, and concentrate on becoming your own nutrition guru. There are hundreds of books available. Acquiring knowledge in an area that's important to you is intoxicating. Each book you read will only increase your passion for learning. Keep an open mind, and do not stop at one source. You can learn at least one thing from each book, even if you don't agree with everything in it.

Food for Thought

To change one's life
Start immediately
Do it flamboyantly
No exceptions
    —William James

No two people are the same in terms of their exercise and nutrition needs. We have varying shapes, sizes, and metabolic rates, so don't worry if someone else's plan is not working for you! We have met hundreds of people, and everyone has his or her idea of the right way to lose weight.

Will this book be the final word on healthy eating? Of course not. Dr. Peter J. D'Adamo said that most of what we know about human nutrition has been attained in the last 100 years, with new studies coming out weekly. The more you know, the more you realize you don't know! Deep down inside, you know what you ought to be doing. The great Roman orator Cicer said, "Nobody can give you wiser advice than yourself."

Start your investigation today and reap the benefits! Keep your eyes and ears open for sound information. And with some trial and error, you will be able to determine what is right. Waiting around for the perfect time to *take action* is simply postponing your right to enjoy good health. And once you get started and are well on your way, you'll probably ask yourself, "Why didn't I start all this sooner?"

Eating healthy and maintaining an exercise program all year round does get easier as time goes on. You don't have to give up your friends, families, and social functions. It takes time to get comfortable with new eating strategies: you have spent many years adapting your body to your current eating habits, so don't expect to make too many changes overnight.

You'll begin to see and feel results in time. It's human nature to want it all *now*. This is the time to reflect on the powerful reasons that inspired you to make those new decisions. Hopefully, these reasons are more powerful than the numbers on the scale. If they aren't, you'll need to re-evaluate why the results have become more important than the reasons.

We know you are excited, but trying to add too many new behaviors at one time can be overwhelming, which makes the entire process tedious. The biggest consequence of setting impossible standards is disappointment, which most often leads to giving up altogether. Gradual changes made with a conscious effort can last a lifetime. And you are worth it.

Health Miracle Activities

1. Do you have any nutrition habits that are not serving you? Be honest and list them now.

   _____

   _____

2. Describe the effects your present eating habits have on your health and energy level.

   _____

   _____

3. What are the benefits you would experience if you made some positive changes?

   _____

   _____

4. Who else in your life would benefit if you made positive changes?

_____

5. What is one strategy from this chapter you will implement today?

_____

6. Close your eyes, take a few deep breaths, then think of your new nutrition strategy. Now picture yourself taking the action step. Smile to yourself and nod your head as you see yourself reaping the benefits. Fast-forward one year and imagine the results.

Chapter 5

*My goal is to remain healthy my entire career, and a
healthy diet seems like a good start.*

—Tiger Woods, pro golf champion

The Miracle of Health Nutrition Recommendations

There is no one right diet for everyone all the time. It is crucial that each person contemplating a change in diet monitor his or her own body's feedback, the feelings it emits of "okay" or "not okay."
—Annemarie Colbin, Ph.D

Think Lifestyle

Instead of a diet (remember, it is a nasty four-letter word), we want to focus on the healthiest foods on the planet, foods that can add vigor to your day, bolster your immune system, and support your desire for a lean, trim physique. No fad diet can meet the needs of every person. We are all different in our genetic makeup, activity levels, metabolic rates, likes and dislikes—the list goes on and on. Factor in the changing requirements of your body as you age and it is impossible to find one diet that will work over the long term.

Instead of providing you with a restriction in calories and an exhaustive nutritional breakdown of food, we would like to share the nutritional secrets of some of the healthiest populations on the planet. Just by choosing better foods and following some of the strategies in the previous chapter, you can reap tremendous health benefits, and you don't need to weigh every item on your plate!

"Tell us what you eat" is the most common request we get during our corporate consultations, so we have included our Top Foods List, the foods you will find in our home. The second most popular question we are asked is, "What should I take?" Read on to learn about our favorite health supplement recommendations that are based on scientific studies and research. You should consider some safe, basic supplements for abundant health. We will share our family's plan with you.

Once you start adapting to a new way of eating—adding more Top Foods and removing "junk" foods, consuming more water, and reducing sugar-laden drinks—then you could check with a natural health care provider, registered dietitian, or holistic nutritionist for further information to make sure that you are meeting all of your nutritional needs.

The Healthiest "Diets" on the Planet

To keep the body in good health is a duty . . . otherwise we shall not be able to keep our mind strong and clear.
—Buddha

Two parts of the world, the Japanese island of Okinawa and the Mediterranean area (including southern Italy, Portugal, Spain, southern France, and Greece), are stellar role models when it comes to nutrition and lifestyle. Both of these areas have some of the healthiest people on the planet, people who live long, energetic, independent lives. The Okinawa population is virtually free from obesity and has a much lower risk for age-related illnesses. Their typical diet is low in salt, trans fats, sugar, and processed foods. Fruits, vegetables, fish, and freshly ground flaxseed are mainstays. Foods are lightly stir-fried with healthy oils, and close to 40 grams of fiber are consumed daily. The typical serving size is less than half of the average North American serving!

The Mediterranean diet is a heart-healthy eating plan endorsed by the Mayo Clinic and supported by many scientific studies. This eating style significantly reduces the risk of further heart disease in individuals who have experienced a heart attack. It is also associated with lower LDL (low-density lipoprotein, the bad cholesterol). The diet includes salads, beans (chickpeas, lentils, split peas, and fava beans), vegetables, whole grains (polenta, couscous, bulgur, rice, and wheat), and fruits. Small portions of lean meat such as lamb, chicken, and beef are popular. Milk products, in the form of natural cheeses and butter, are used sparingly as condiments. There are very few processed foods, and dry red wine is consumed in small amounts. Herbs and spices are abundant and only quality fats are consumed: olive oil, fish, avocados, flaxseeds, walnuts, and sunflower seeds.

Both the Okinawa and Mediterranean people average 9 hours of sleep per night and enjoy active lifestyles and close family ties—the best results for a body makeover are always gained through a combination of exercise, nutrition, and healthy lifestyle practices. Our favorite experts, including health guru Dr. Andrew Weil and Canadian researcher Sam Graci, endorse the Okinawa and Mediterranean lifestyles.

According to the National Heart, Lung, and Blood Institute, about one in three adults in the United States have high blood pressure (hypertension) as of April 2008. Exercise, in combination with diet modifications, is the most effective treatment. The DASH diet (Dietary Approaches to Stop Hypertension) recommends a diet rich in vegetables, fruits, and low-fat dairy products. The diet also limits sodium intake and alcohol. The National Institute of Health and the Mayo Clinic recommend this dietary guideline for lowering hypertension.

Go Organic

I don't eat junk food and I don't think junk thoughts.
　　—Peace Pilgrim, peace activist

For those of you who are ready to take your eating experience to a new level, try switching some of your favorite foods to the organic version. Being very healthy to begin with, we couldn't imagine how eating organic food would make that much of a difference for us, but we are always willing to try new things and our research into organic foods was perking our interest. Over a four-year period, we slowly switched to mostly organic foods. Some of the significant benefits we have personally noticed are: fewer cravings and less overeating; an easier time in maintaining ideal weight; and a reclaiming of our intuitive sense of what is good for our bodies.

There is still a lot of debate about the nutritional differences between nonorganic and organic foods. At the very least, if you choose organic foods, you will avoid the pesticides, herbicides, and fungicides that are used in conventional farming. Purchase organic to reduce this toxic load for your family and your environment. You can start by choosing the organic versions of the following foods as they are the top 10 most heavily sprayed: pears, grapes, apples, spinach, strawberries, green beans, celery, lettuce, wheat, and peaches.

Hydrate for Health

I believe that water is the only drink for a wise man.
—Henry David Thoreau

What do scientists look for when they explore a planet's ability to support human life? Do they look for a good Italian restaurant? No! They look for water. Water supports life as we know it. Water is one of the essential nutrients. Essential means mandatory—it's not an option if you want to have great health over the course of a lifetime. After reading the next few pages, you might be inspired to get yourself a glass of water.

Water is foundational for all the important biochemical reactions in the body. Like a wilted houseplant, your body will respond to water immediately. Science has demonstrated that increasing your water intake has positive effects on your energy levels, can help you shed excess pounds, and may help fight certain types of cancers. Water is one of the true miraculous elixirs of life.

Your blood is 95 percent water. Muscle is about 70 percent water. The human fetus at three months is 90 percent water, as reported in the *Journal of Biological Chemistry*. A 45-year-old man would be about 65 percent water, while a 70-year-old man is only 43 percent water. It is imperative that you continue to rehydrate your cells as much as possible with water. It is the most important thing you can do for your complexion besides getting a good night's sleep. Drinking more water should be near the top of your to-do list each day. Dr. Batmanghelidj, in his book *Your Body's Many Cries for Water*, reported there are people in North America who may be mistaking the symptoms of dehydration for those of being ill. Don't wait until you feel thirsty to enjoy a glass of water.

If you are dehydrated, your body will scavenge water from your skin, the mucous membranes in your nose, and your eyes to maintain equilibrium in the cells of your body. Your joints are yet another victim. The moist synovial linings, cartilage, and disks all take a beating in the body of the chronically dehydrated. Is that news for any of you suffering from arthritis pain or lower back pain?

What else do you need to know about water? A 1 percent loss of water will affect brain function; a 2 percent decrease will cause you to notice physical changes. Allow yourself to be dehydrated by 2 or 3 percent and you will lose 25 percent of your overall efficiency. If you were stranded in the wild, this could mean life or death. Why put yourself at risk when water is readily available? Your body needs water for:

Thermoregulation: Your beautiful body needs water to maintain its ideal temperature.

Cardiac function: Your amazing heart beats about 86,000 times a day. It has to work harder when you are dehydrated.

Digestion: If you knew how many products were sold in supermarkets and drugstores to help people with digestive issues, you would run for a glass of water right this very moment. Many people are constipated and feel the side effects of being *plugged up.* Did you know that one function of the large intestine and colon is the uptake of water? If your cells are dehydrated, your bowels are one of the first places your body goes to scavenge for water, leading to harder stool that sits stagnant in your colon. Are you thinking what we are thinking? Breath mint anyone?

Your blood: Liz Applegate, Ph.D., says that dehydrated blood moves more slowly because it becomes sticky and thick, so there will be less oxygen and nutrients moving into your cells.

Earth-friendly Green Tip

One billion plastic water bottles are thrown out per week in America. Seventy-six percent are not recycled.

It takes over 1,000 years for a plastic water bottle to decompose. Try using an eco-friendly steel one!

New York Times best-selling author, Dr. Masaru Emoto, in his book, *The Miracle of Water*, wrote that the water in your body responds to your thoughts and feelings. Imagine you have a fresh lemon in one hand and a sharp knife in the other. Take the knife and cut that sour lemon right down the middle. Bring one of the halves up close to your nose and inhale its fragrance. Now imagine biting into it and having the juice run down your chin. Is your mouth watering?

Can you see how our words affected your body's response? Your mouth watered and it was only from an imagined event. Your thoughts do affect your body! And the effects are almost immediate. You can alter the physiological state of your body just by changing the thoughts you are thinking!

Emoto's incredible experiments involved freezing water in containers that had either been labeled with certain words or meditated on by a group of people. Some of the labels and meditations were very positive, while others were very negative. The water was frozen and the resulting water crystals examined under a high-power microscope. Miraculously, one container had beautifully formed crystals, while the other container had deformed crystals. You can guess which container received the positive labels and meditations! Now you can put new meaning to the words: "Worry yourself sick."

Hopefully, by now you are thinking that you should drink more water, so how much do you need? You often hear eight glasses per day. Once again, it really depends on your age, activity level, size, and other factors. One formula that takes some individual differences into account is:

$$\frac{\text{Body weight in pounds}}{2} = \text{number of ounces per day}$$

For a 150-pound woman:

$$\frac{150}{2} = 75 \text{ ounces of water (or nine 8-ounce cups per day)}$$

This formula was designed by holistic health care practitioner Paul Check. It is intended to give you an amount of water for superior health. In Paul's own words: "The solution for pollution is dilution." Start by increasing one cup at a time until you reach your optimal level of water. Give yourself the gift of feeling and looking better with fresher breath, healthier skin, brighter eyes, better digestion, and increased energy.

If you switched one of the beverages you drank during the day to water, you would decrease your caloric intake by at least 100 calories (i.e., the amount of calories in a cup of orange juice). If this was the only change you made in your diet, you could lose 6–9 pounds in one year, so don't drink your calories!

Health Miracle

Researchers at the Fred Hutchinson Research Center in Seattle found that the risk of colon cancer decreased in half for the women in the study who drank a minimum of eight glasses of water per day.

Health Miracle Top Foods Nutrition Plan

The biggest seller is cookbooks and the second is diet books—how not to eat what you've just learned how to cook.
—Andy Rooney, humorist and commentator

The average person eats from the same list of 12 foods day after day, week after week. Food psychologist Brian Wansink says "Every single one of us eats how much we eat largely because of what's around us." And many of the foods you are ingesting on a regular basis are heavily processed, full of bad fats, refined carbohydrates, and are certainly not serving your health. But great marketing, attractive labels, and availability of these unhealthy foods allow us to mindlessly overeat and suffer the consequences.

A simple way to change your eating habits without counting calories is to make better food choices available to your family by adopting our Top Foods Nutrition Plan. We have provided you with a list of the best possible foods for your health. These foods come from our studies of the healthiest people on the planet mentioned in the previous section. The foods are jam-packed with nutrients and are guaranteed to enhance your wellness. The plan is simple. Look over the following list and pick one item to add to your current diet. At the same time, take a good look at your cupboards and refrigerator and eliminate one food that is not serving you (high sugar, high fat, low nutritional value). If you need some help to get started, we have chosen foods from the Top Foods list that are champions. Read on to find the Top Food Champions you should start with. We have also provided a list of the most detrimental items, the Furious Four Cell Destroyers. These should be cut down or eliminated first. Every two to three weeks, repeat this strategy and you will eventually find yourself eating more nutrient-dense foods. This will automatically reduce your cravings, calories, and urges to overeat, giving you quick results with increased energy and fat loss. The best part is you won't have to fight the emotional upheaval common in popular restriction diets.

Health Miracle

Green tea has strong antioxidant properties and it can give you a high level of alertness without the ups and downs of other caffeinated beverages. It is an ideal performance drink!

Health Miracle Top Foods List

Beverages: Green tea, organic wines, water

Condiments: Extra-virgin olive oil (first cold-pressed), turmeric spice, sea salt

Dairy: Plain organic yogurt

Fruits: Cherries, prunes, oranges, blueberries, raspberries, strawberries, avocados, apples, tomatoes, bananas, plums, oranges, grapefruit, kiwi

Grains: Brown rice, steel-cut oatmeal, spelt, kamut, millet cereals, brown rice pasta, brown rice wraps

Meat and alternatives: Organic free-range chicken and beef, organic eggs, wild Pacific salmon, kidney beans, tilapia, halibut, Mahi tuna

Nuts and seeds: Raw almonds, sunflower seeds, freshly ground flax-seeds, raw walnuts, raw cashews, raw pumpkin seeds

> *Vegetables:* Broccoli, cauliflower, peppers (green/orange/red/yellow), celery, cucumber, carrots, yams, spinach, asparagus, a variety of squash, beets, bok choy, kale, garlic, and onions

Some Top Food Champions

Berries: We recommend 1 cup daily of fresh or frozen berries.

Fruits and vegetables: Fruits and vegetables are some of the richest nutrient powerhouses of the food groups. Including them in your daily intake is one of the keys to a treasure chest of vitality.

> *For some of our favorite recipes, visit our Web site: www.FitSpeakers.com*

Plant food provides a rich source of antioxidants and phytochemicals, substances that have many health-protective benefits. They have been linked with the prevention and/or treatment of heart disease, cancer, diabetes, and a host of other medical conditions. Research has shown that people who consume 5 to 10 servings of fruits and vegetables have *half the risk* of developing cancer. And if they do get cancer, their chances of dying are lower. Fruits and vegetables are also naturally low in cholesterol and sodium, which are linked to heart disease.

Garlic and onions: Dr. Tieraona Low Dog, director of education for the Program in Integrative Medicine at the University of Arizona, reported that men who eat an abundance of garlic and onions have less risk of prostate cancer. *Note:* Cooking garlic takes away much of its medicinal properties. Try freshly crushed garlic, lemon, and oil on veggies and whole grain rice. It's also great in vinaigrettes.

Salmon and other omega-3 fats: There is so much to say about this Food Champion that we have created an entire section called "Increase Your Healthy Fats" further on in this chapter.

Turmeric: Known for its use in curry, turmeric has an anti-inflammatory effect in the body. Johns Hopkins Hospital conducted a study that showed a 66 percent reduction of polyps (abnormal growth or tumor) in the intestines after six months of supplementation with 1 teaspoon of turmeric per day.

> ### *Health Miracle*
>
> **There is a phytonutrient compound in berries called pterostilbene. Dr. Agnes Rimando, Ph.D., reports that this compound is more effective than some drugs at reducing elevated cholesterol levels.**

The Furious Four Cell Destroyers

Highly processed foods: Yes, we are talking about all the convenient foods that are manufactured to make your life a little easier. Too bad they come with health consequences. Harvard Medical School researchers confirm that resistance to insulin can be doubled by eating fast foods twice per week. Insulin resistance is a precursor to diabetes. People who regularly eat refined foods (e.g., high-sugar breakfast cereals, fast foods, frozen dinners, white rice, refined pastas, candy bars, and white bread) will be missing many nutrients in their diets, leaving them fatigued and compromising their overall health. According to Dr. Loren Cordain in the 2005 *American Journal of Clinical Nutrition*, processed foods "negatively affect proximate factors, which underlie or worsen chronic diseases in civilization."

Salt: Reduce or eliminate the amount of table salt you consume. White table salt is processed and contains ingredients you do not need. Most people are taking in more than they need if they are eating processed foods and packaged or canned foods. Too much salt increases water retention and the risk of high blood pressure. If you cook your own meals and rarely eat processed foods, you may add some salt—a small amount is necessary for many cell functions. The natural form is sea salt. We sprinkle a pinch on our main meals to taste. We use Nature's Cargo Traditional Coarse Grey Sea Salts from France.

Sugar: Reduce or eliminate refined sugar in your diet. Too much sugar leads to obesity, diabetes, roller-coaster energy levels, and a number of other conditions. In the 1850s we ate only 3–4 pounds of sugar in a year, but now that average has increased to over 130 pounds annually, all consumed in a variety of forms: table sugar or sucrose, corn syrup, corn sweetener, barley malt, dextrose, galactose, fructose, and maltose. You have to become a sugar detective! Processed foods and canned soda are the key culprits. Sugar is a preservative that also enhances flavor, so you will find it in everything from french fries to hamburger buns.

Trans fats: Brad King, in *Fat Wars*, calls these the "Frankenstein Fats." These fats have been transformed through a chemical process called hydrogenation, which increases food's shelf life and makes the altered fats easier to integrate into the cells of your body. It's reported that they cause chaos and confusion in your cells. Trans fats raise the level of LDL, the unhealthy cholesterol, and they decrease HDL (high-density lipoprotein), the healthy cholesterol, increasing your chances of coronary heart disease. According to some scientists, the heart disease epidemic may be partly due to the increase of trans fats in our Western diet.

Frequently consumed foods that contain trans fats are stick margarine, shortening, fast foods, chips and crackers, doughnuts, frozen foods (waffles and fish sticks), some breakfast cereals and granola bars, toppings, dips, non-dairy coffee creamers, soup cups, and many store-bought baked goods. Remember to avoid these foods and any others with labels containing the words "hydrogenated" and "partially hydrogenated." The U.S. Department of Agriculture and the U.S. Department of Health and Human Services Guidelines recommend keeping consumption of trans fatty acids as low as possible.

> **Did You Know?**
> *The U. S. National Heart, Lung, and Blood Institute reports that drinking more than one soft drink per day, whether regular or diet, increases the risk of metabolic syndrome by more than 40 percent.*

Increase Your Healthy Fats

Your body will not perform well without these necessary fats. They have a direct impact, keeping your skin looking young, sustaining a healthy heart, maintaining healthy hair, and promoting keen mental concentration. The healthy fats are essential to life. They are necessary for healing and repair, and they are an integral part of our cell walls. Fats are essential for brain and nervous system development and they play an important part in hormonal regulation. Fats are even needed for the absorption of some vitamins. And for athletes, they are necessary for optimal performance. We will concentrate on the best fats you can add to your diet without getting too technical on you. Here are the food sources that can add these essential fats to your diet. Later in this chapter, we will share the supplements that we use to ensure our optimal intake of omega-3 fats.

Omega-3 fats are essential to your diet. There are two ways to get them: from plant sources or from fish sources. You need both types for well-rounded nutrition as they provide different benefits.

Plant sources are freshly ground flaxseeds, walnuts, soybeans, and leafy greens. We are frequently asked if flax oil is a good option. It is better to think of it as another form of healthy fat that you can use as a condiment, but the oil lacks the antioxidant-rich lignans and the fiber that you get from the ground flaxseed, so it is worthwhile to invest in a grinder and grind your own flaxseeds each morning. You can purchase ground flaxseed, but nothing beats freshly ground!

Fish sources have received much attention for their link to a variety of health benefits. They have been shown to decrease clot and plaque formation, protect against irregular heartbeat, decrease triglycerides, lower blood pressure, reduce inflammation and joint tenderness, and are even linked to a decrease in cognitive decline and depression. There is a huge concern over the contaminants found in our fish today, so this is one area where we choose to supplement our diet. We have chosen a high-quality fish oil supplement that has been filtered to remove impurities and contaminants like mercury. Read to the end of this chapter for the brand we prefer.

Extra-virgin olive oil is another form of fat full of antioxidants that should be included in your daily diet. Use it to replace butter or as a part of a healthy salad dressing (1–2 tablespoons per day is a healthy dose). This is the fat that is abundant in the Mediterranean diet. These countries are known to have very low rates of heart disease, and science has shown a reduction in bad cholesterol (LDL) and an increase in good cholesterol (HDL) in people who substitute unhealthy fats with monounsaturated fats like olive oil. Look for a first cold-pressed (organic if possible) oil to get the best possible quality. Other mono-unsaturated fats are avocados and nuts, which are great on salads or as part of a healthy snack.

Health Miracle

Even the American Medical Association recommends that every person at risk of heart disease consume omega-3s. In 2006 a group of researchers found that increased consumption of omega-3 fatty acids from fish or fish oil supplements (but not from ALA [alpha-linolenic acid] sources) reduced the rates of all-cause mortality, cardiac and sudden death, and possible stroke.

Supplements

What is the most confusing topic on the planet? Some think the World Wide Web. Others might say, "The stock market." We would answer, "The supplement section of the nutrition store or supermarket." The shelves are loaded with hundreds of colorful containers filled with powders, pills, capsules, and liquids. To the uninformed, novice health enthusiast, it looks overwhelming. Even to the experienced athlete, it can be confusing! They all claim they have benefits and each of them says they have active ingredients.

A supplement is any mineral, vitamin, amino acid, herb, or dietary substance used to increase total nutrient intake. As you can see, this definition includes a wide range of products. Our focus in this chapter is to increase your awareness about supplements and to provide you with some sound advice when it comes to making your own decisions about supplementing your diet.

Many people think health and fitness can be bought and paid for in a pill. We believe that for optimum health, you must first maximize your nourishment from whole food sources. Secondly, you must include daily physical activity, incorporating cardiovascular, flexibility, and resistance-type activities into every week. Thirdly, adequate sleep of at least 7 hours per night is necessary for health and vitality. Fourthly, practise relaxation techniques to counteract daily stresses and promote a stronger immune system. We have included several of these techniques in Chapter 11. Your supplement regime should be the icing on the cake, the insurance that you are doing the best for yourself and your family. Always enlist the help of a health care practitioner to help you navigate through the supplement maze!

According to the *Journal of the American Medical Association* (JAMA), the following people could benefit from a daily multivitamin/mineral:

- those who do not eat at least five servings of vegetables and fruits per day
- those who do not consume fish on a weekly basis
- people on a low-calorie, weight-loss diet
- vegetarians and vegans
- people over 60
- women in their childbearing years
- people who are lactose intolerant or have food allergies
- people with a family history of cancer or heart disease

Eight Reasons to Use Supplements

Yes, definitely, you require vitamin supplements, antioxidant supplements, mineral supplements and medicinal herbal supplements to help your body and mind withstand the extreme stress and pressure of a faster-is-better, 24-7-365 society.
—Sam Graci

1. **To eliminate nutritional deficiencies:** Everyone ought to eat the best-quality food available. However, this can be difficult in our fast-paced world. With many men and women working outside of the home, little time and energy is left for food preparation. Fast foods, as well as heavily refined and processed foods, have become a staple for many families. The problem? Nutrients are leached out of these foods during processing from field to market! Throw in the additives and preservatives, and your food no longer serves you when it comes to your health.

2. **To get enough vitamin, mineral, essential fat, and antioxidant support for our unique needs:** Our nutritional needs

are not the same. It's naive to take the recommended dose of any vitamin or supplement and assume you're getting enough for your own health benefits. Some of us may require more, others less. Only through careful study and consultation with your health care practitioner can you determine if you are meeting your own needs.

3. **To fight free radicals:** Some supplements have an antioxidant effect. This means they counteract the damage done to the body by environmental pollutants (such as smog and cigarette smoke) and by the body's natural waste production.

4. **To aid in excess fat loss:** Dr. Joey Shulman, in her book *The Last 15*, claims that replacing saturated fats with fish oil supplements can aid in the reduction of abdominal fat. This is based on recent scientific research, unlike many fat-loss supplement claims.

5. **To increase energy levels:** Vitamins and other nutrients are necessary for the energy-producing reactions in the human cell. An organic, whole-foods diet, combined with an exemplary life-style, can meet most of these needs, but how many of us are living this way? Depending on individual needs, supplementation may be necessary for more energy.

6. **To assist elite athletes:** Some athletes train at high intensities for prolonged hours, depleting their stores of nutrients. Several sports require extra protein, and traveling athletes could benefit from increased immune support through supplementation.

7. **To support graceful aging:** In their groundbreaking work, *You: The Owner's Manual*, Dr. Oz and Dr. Roizen say, "The correct multivitamin taken twice a day can make your RealAge more than six years younger."

8. **To reduce the risk of illness:** It has been shown that certain supplements may help to fight and reduce many diseases. Hundreds of studies have shown that fish oil supplementation can act as an

anti-inflammatory agent in the body. It is especially protective for the heart and has been shown to reduce the risk of heart attack dramatically.

Health Miracle

In a study done in Australia, participants experienced a 71 percent reduced risk of sudden cardiac death due to irregular heart rhythms after only four weeks of fish oil supplementation.

One rule we like to follow is to add only one new supplement at a time to our nutritional regimen. This way we can determine if there are any positive, noticeable benefits or undesirable side effects. Even though many products are called "all natural," there can be ingredients that may have an adverse effect on your system. It's ironic that supplements are under so much scrutiny when every year thousands of people who don't use them die prematurely from misusing food (e.g., obesity-related diseases).

On a positive note, supplements can become an important part of the daily ritual of self-care. Taking supplements at the same time every day can help you to habitualize the action, like brushing your teeth in the morning. By continually making a commitment to improvement, you can make small advances in your life that could take you to a new level each time.

One of the most powerful impacts of supplements is the psychological effect of doing a little more than the average person. When you know you have spent some time, energy, and money on achieving your fitness goals, you are more likely to take your efforts seriously.

Uche's Story

I remember being given cod-liver oil by my mother when I was very young. It's funny now to think back and remember the disgusted look on my brothers' and sisters' faces when we knew it was TIME.

My mother would bring out this large, funny-looking silver spoon after breakfast. Because of the size of the spoon, we were never quite able to get the entire amount of the thick, room-temperature oil into our mouths. The result? Whoever went last would get a lot of backwash!

Well, looking back with what I know now about essential fats, our mother was right on track and a great role model. If you were to peek into our refrigerator or kitchen cupboards today, you would see the influence of my mother's early guidance.

Our General Health Supplement Choices

We did not provide an exhaustive list of supplements for you to read through. Our objective was to stir a desire on your part to take ownership of your health, to do some investigation on your own, and make the commitment to take your health and fitness to the next level. The following are the foundation of our supplements. Most people should consider a fish oil, a probiotic, and a multivitamin. We also use specific supplements that have been personalized for our own nutritional needs from our naturopathic doctor.

Genuine Health (www.genuinehealth.com)
Tel: 416-977-3505 Toll-free: 877-500-7888

Our favorite products from Genuine Health:

greens+ kids — A colorful blend of organic fruits and vegetables— with additional ingredients such as probiotics—for your children.

greens+ multi+ — A high potency complete multivitamin/ mineral plus green+, a unique blend of over 23 plant-based ingredients providing essential nutrients and antioxidants.

nutrilean+ express bar — A nutritious and delicious 100 percent natural meal replacement bar with the perfect balance of healthy carbohydrates, fiber, and protein, plus 24 essential vitamins and minerals.

o3mega — A superior source of research-proven omega-3 fatty acids derived from pure, wild, and sustainable fish oils that are enteric coated, ensuring maximum absorption and no fishy repeat.

proteins+ — The most advanced and bio-available alpha+™ whey protein isolate.

Genestra Brands (www.seroyal.com)

Multivitamins and minerals — Genestra offers specific multivitamins and minerals for pregnancy, children, etc.

Super HMF powder — A probiotic supplement that helps stimulate growth of the friendly, healthy bacteria that reside in our digestive system; this is especially important if you are taking antibiotics, which destroy bad and good bacteria.

Supplement Safety

www.consumerlab.com: Independent lab that tests supplements for potency and purity

www.ifos.com: International Fish Oil Standards at the University of Guelph, a Web site for analyzing fish oil supplements for contaminants or impurities

www.nccam.nci.nih.gov/health: U.S. National Institute of Health's National Center for Complementary and Alternative Medicine has the latest FDA danger alerts, the latest research on drug interactions, and more

www.crnusa.org: Council for Responsible Nutrition

http://ods.od.nih.gov: U.S. Office of Dietary Supplements

Health Miracle Activities

1. Write down the foods from our Top Foods List that you regularly include in your diet:

   _____

2. What new foods will you try in the next month?

   _____

3. Which supplements will you investigate after reading this chapter?

   _____

Chapter 6

Physical fitness is the first requisite of happiness. It is the attainment of a uniformly developed body as well as a sound mind, fully capable of naturally, easily, and satisfactorily performing our many and varied daily tasks with spontaneous zest and pleasure.

—Joseph Pilates

Goodbye Fat, Hello Fitness!

Exercise is that good for you. You name just about any health problem, and you'll find that exercise helps prevent it or cure it. Exercise is the elixir of life.
　—Liz Applegate, Ph.D.

This is undoubtedly one of our favorite chapters in this book. Why? Because we have collected and compiled revolutionary, scientific proof that exercise is paramount to your long-term physical, mental, and emotional health. Exercise is a modern-day miracle: It helps to prevent heart disease, stroke, diabetes, obesity, and even cancer. It will make your bones stronger, improve your blood lipid profile (cholesterol and fats in the blood), increase your strength, and restore your balance. Exercise stimulates new blood vessel growth in your brain, heart, and skeletal muscle, increasing the amount of oxygen and nutrients to these areas. It can help regulate appetite, increase attention span, boost energy, improve sleep quality, and generally make you feel better.

If medical doctors could write a prescription for exercise, they would. As we write these words, medical researchers are scurrying to find a pharmaceutical equivalent to the hormone leptin, which naturally increases in your body with regular physical activity. Why leptin? Well, this is the hormone that inhibits appetite. It will likely be many years before science can duplicate what the body does naturally, so get moving!

This chapter is loaded with reasons to *take action!* We guarantee that you will feel the urge to get your arms and legs moving after reading it. Maybe even while reading!

> **Health Miracle**
>
> In 2007, German researchers conducted a human study that tested participants on vocabulary words before and after exercise sessions. The rate of learning increased by 20 percent after exercise!

From Your Seat to Your Feet!

When health is absent
Wisdom cannot reveal itself,
Art cannot be exerted,
Wealth is useless and Reason is powerless.
    —Herophilies

We have become a nation that sits—in our cars, at work, at home, and even at play with our home computer games. Hypokinesis (*hypo:* under or less; *kinesis:* motion or activity) is a condition that affects millions of North Americans who do not make time for regular exercise. It amazes us to see how few people even make it outside for the occasional walk. There are days we have been out in our community and not seen another person, yet we are literally surrounded by thousands of houses! "Where is everyone?" is a question that we frequently ask each other even though we both know the answer: the lure of home computers, video games, television, and the almighty La-Z-Boy recliner is hard to resist. Hypokinesis has a ripple effect in many areas—how you feel, how you look, how you sleep, how you age, how you perform daily tasks, and even how well your brain functions.

Did you know that the average person spends 80–90 percent of the time indoors?

You have approximately 640 muscles and 206 bones in that incredible body of yours that were designed for movement. If you don't use them, you lose them! Inactivity also makes your circulatory (blood) and lymphatic (immune) systems stagnant and your breathing shallow. When this happens, your brain gets less fuel;

yawning becomes a last-ditch effort to increase the flow of oxygen to your 18 billion brain cells.

People often associate the word "exercise" with sacrifice and pain. The minute they even hear the word, they conjure up images of spending less time with their family and friends, giving up freedom, and spending incredible amounts of money on gym memberships, workout wear, and personal trainers. Many people have an *all-or-nothing* attitude that immobilizes them or postpones their movement toward health and happiness. These thinking patterns are usually strongly rooted and challenging to change.

Some people will wait until they manifest a health tragedy or set-back before they decide to take action. In this chapter it is our intention to rekindle or reinforce your desire to make fitness a priority in your life by sharing with you some of the most powerful research that conclusively proves exercise can have a positive impact on every area of your life.

James's Story

A man ran up to us in our conference room in Seattle. He told us that he had been at our seminar the year before and had since turned his life around. "I was on a slow path to obesity and an eventual self-inflicted gunshot wound called a heart attack. My grandmother always told me that most men in our family die young from complications of cardiovascular disease. I decided: Not this man! I am on a path of healthy foods, great times, and newfound joy in fitness. I started just by doing push-ups and sit-ups when I got home after your presentation last year."

The following year, James e-mailed us a picture of himself skiing down Mount Hood with his son, leaner, happier, and full of enthusiasm for life!

Health Miracle

In our Western society, a decline in health typically starts during the third decade of life. By the time the average person has reached 70, he or she has lost 30 percent of strength, 15–30 percent of bone mass, 60 percent of maximal breathing capacity, and 40 percent of kidney and liver function. Regular exercise can *radically* lower all of these percentages.

A "Neat" Way to Get Started

There are risks and costs to a program of action. But they are far less than the long-range risks and costs of comfortable inaction.
—John F. Kennedy

The April 2008 issue of *Nutrition Action Healthletter* included an interview with James Levine, endocrinologist and professor of medicine at the Mayo Clinic in Rochester, where he heads up a lab called the NEAT lab. We were intrigued by his research in non-exercise activity thermogenesis (NEAT). This involves any movement not specifically done for the purpose of physical fitness (i.e., gardening, walking, shopping, cleaning, etc.). His research concluded that non-exercising obese people move an average of 2.5 hours less per day than non-exercising lean people. If you aren't eager to join a gym, then you may want to consider upping your daily NEAT expenditure to get your motor started and burn off some of that stored body fat. Here are some things to try:

- Pace while you talk on the phone.
- Ride an exercise bike while you watch TV in the comfort of your own home.
- Get up for a stretch and a small glass of water during commercial breaks.
- Look for the farthest parking spots instead of the closest ones.
- Use the stairs instead of the elevator or escalator.
- Start a garden and take care of it yourself.
- Wash the car by hand.
- Offer to help a neighbor with some yard work.
- Redecorate an area of your house or move some furniture around each week.
- Throw away all your remote controls.

Health Miracle

Northern Gas Company employees took 80 percent fewer sick days while participating in a corporate exercise program.

Boost Your Productivity

The power of exercise seems far more impressive than that of brain-training software.
      —Sandra Aamodt

Can you imagine being more productive at home and at work? Can you imagine fewer illnesses and increased immunity for your entire family? Well, stop imagining! Lace up your sneakers and put on your exercise gear! The *International Journal of Sports Medicine* reported that immune cells remain elevated for about 3 hours after a 45-minute walk. In 2004 researchers at Leeds Metropolitan University in England studied 210 participants who used their company's gym for aerobics, weight training, or yoga classes during their lunch breaks. The workers demonstrated more productivity and reported they were better able to handle their workloads. They also felt less stress and fatigue in the afternoon.

> *Check out the Web site www.smallstep.gov for more great tips to increase your daily activity.*

Health Miracle

General Electric reported that members of the company fitness center decreased their medical claims by 27 percent; Coca-Cola published a report that health care claims had lowered by $500 for each employee involved in the company's fitness program; NASA had a 12.5 percent boost in productivity by fitness program participants; and Johnson & Johnson reduced their absenteeism rate by 15 percent within two years of the implementation of a wellness program!

Fitness and the Brain

Exercise is the single most powerful tool you have to optimize your brain function. . . .
      —Dr. John Ratey

We were still buzzing with the energy of our speaking engagement to 800 people in Denver as we rushed through the airport to catch our flight back to Toronto. We paused to pick up some reading material in a bookstore. You can imagine our excitement when we happened to see a cartoon of a brain pumping weights on the front cover of the February 2008 *U.S. News & World Report*. The headline read: "Keeping Your Brain Fit: The Latest Science on Boosting Your Memory and Protecting against Alzheimer's." Fitness fanatics that we are, we quickly flipped the magazine open and were thrilled to see in bold letters: **Sound body, sound mind.** So much for the term "dumb jock"!

In 2007, researchers at Columbia University showed increased blood flow to a part of the brain responsible for memory after only three months of regular exercise. The participants also experienced faster reaction times and better ability to focus. Exercise stimulates growth factor proteins, which are key to the growth and formation of neural synapses and brain cells. The article also mentioned an exciting new study by British scientists in which people who exercised around 200 minutes per week had chromosome tips (which shorten with age) as long as sedentary people up to 10 years younger. Exercise is antiaging for the brain!

Another study in 2007 had adults aged 50–64 perform a 35-minute treadmill session at between 60–70 percent of maximum heart rate. A control group watched a movie. Both groups were tested on cognitive function after the 35 minutes and no change was observed in the movie watchers, but the runners improved their processing speed and cognitive flexibility after just one workout. This would make a great case for a lunch-hour aerobic workout if you were planning to ask for a pay raise in the afternoon!

Do you need more proof? Then read on!

Henry Lodge, the coauthor of *Younger Next Year*, says that the chemical makeup of your blood will change for most of the day after you exercise. This positive chemical change promotes the regeneration of cells in the body and the brain. Who says exercise can't be a gift that keeps on giving?

Carl Cottman, director of the Institute for Brain Aging and Dementia at the University of California, Irvine, found a direct link between cognitive function and movement in his research. He showed that exercise increases brain-derived neurotrophic factor (BDNF), which is a chemical that helps to build and maintain the neuron connections in the brain.

He was inspired to research BDNF when he noticed in a study on aging that people with the least cognitive decline had three things in common: exercise, education, and self-efficacy. Doesn't this fact make you want to read a good book the next time you are riding a stationary bike?

Neuroscientist Arthur Kramer did research before and after six months of exercise intervention with 60–72-year-old participants. A control group did a stretching routine and the exercise group performed three 1-hour cardiovascular sessions per week. The exercise group experienced a significant improvement in their lungs' ability to process oxygen, but the amazing findings came from the MRI scans of the brain: the exercising group had frontal and temporal brain lobe volume increases!

If you are looking for the best activities to stimulate the brain, get yourself a pair of dancing shoes! John Ratey, Ph.D., in his years of studying fitness and the brain, proved that aerobic exercise is excellent for the brain, but the best way to take advantage of all the benefits is to combine aerobic activity with a sport or activity that challenges the brain. He states: "The more complex the movements, the more complex the synaptic connections."

Choose complex aerobic activities like dancing, cardio classes with choreography, and figure skating. Or combine an aerobic warm-up with rock climbing, gymnastics, yoga, ballet, Pilates, and karate to get the most benefits for your cardiovascular and brain health.

Health Miracle

In 2006 researchers at the University of Illinois conducted a study in which aerobic exercisers increased their brain size by about 3 percent!

Fitness and Your Children

Only 9% of Canadian children and youth (age 5–19) meet the recommended guidelines in Canada's Physical Activity Guides.
　　—www.ParticipACTION.com

Never in the history of the planet have there been so many overweight, unfit kids. Our children are now at risk of developing diseases that were historically seen only in adults. Budget cuts have hit school-based physical education programs hard. Computers and television sets keep kids out of the parks and playgrounds. The rate of obesity among schoolchildren is about six times higher than in 1980.

Exercise can provide some relief for those who suffer with ADHD (attention-deficit hyperactivity disorder). Studies have indicated that complex sports requiring focus (e.g., gymnastics and martial arts) are great for kids who are experiencing the symptoms of ADHD. If your child has been diagnosed with this condition, don't lose hope! Exercise and nutrition can help to balance and harmonize the body and brain.

Tired, overweight, and stressed parents rank fitness low on their priority lists. They don't realize that fitness can have a positive impact on their children's behavior, appearance, self-esteem, and—*yes!*—their academic performance!

In 2008, John Ratey, a psychiatrist, wrote an entire book about exercise and the human brain. He reported that exercise improves learning in three ways: "First it optimizes your mind-set to improve alertness, attention, and motivation; second, it prepares and encourages nerve cells to bind to one another, which is the cellular basis for logging in new information; and third, it spurs the development of new nerve cells from stem cells in the hippocampus." The hippocampus plays a major role in short-term memory and it is one of the first regions of the brain to suffer damage in Alzheimer's disease. Exercise has a protective effect for this area.

Health Miracle

The California Department of Education has been studying the impact of fitness and has repeatedly shown that students with higher fitness scores achieve higher test scores!

The List of Benefits Continues!

The role of exercise has been shown to be consequential in lowering both systolic and diastolic blood pressure. Both aerobic and resistance training have been shown to facilitate anti-hypertensive responses.
—Dr. Len Kravitz

✓ Regular exercise is one of the best things you can do to keep body fat at a healthy level. We have a natural tendency to store fat. One theory explains that people accumulated fat in preparation for famines over the early part of human history. This was great if you were a cave dweller or medieval peasant, but when was the last time your family suffered a famine? Fortunately, we can fool this survival mechanism by staying active. Daily activity tells our cells that there will be a constant supply of nutrients. The cells get the message, metabolism stays high, and food is metabolized for fuel efficiently.

✓ Surveys of women show that exercise helps to alleviate the symptoms experienced before and after menstruation. Women who exercise often report less pain, and they also score better on evaluations of mood and concentration. When it's "that time of the month," head to the gym instead of the chocolate shop!

✓ With resistance training, your muscles and connective tissues become thicker and stronger. This will aid in strength and joint protection. One of our seminar participants swore that her great fitness level not only saved her life, but allowed her to thrive after a near-fatal car accident and months of rehabilitation.

✓ Exercise elevates mood. Endorphins get released from your "inner pharmacy" during exercise. Endorphins, known as nature's opiates—your body's drug of choice—put you in a euphoric state. This is the positive addiction that many people who exercise experience.

✓ Mitochondria are the energy centers of your cells. They produce energy by breaking down fat and carbohydrates. Your marvelous body will multiply the number of mitochondria in your muscle cells as you become fit, adding more energy for your day.

✓ Stretching will increase circulation and warm joints and muscle fibers. Better flexibility and range of motion are important for everyday tasks. Have you ever seen someone whose inflexibility prevented him or her from picking up an object from the floor? How about watching that same person get up off a soft, comfortable chair? With a loud grunt, he or she completes the task—it almost hurts to watch.

Stretching is one of the easiest, cheapest ways to quickly improve your mobility and reduce pain.

✓ Weight-bearing exercise has been shown to prevent bone-density loss. In fact, it's the number-one way to enjoy the confidence of having strong, healthy bones! Hippocrates, in 300 BC, said, "Extreme remedies are appropriate for extreme diseases." Prevention is always better than dealing with the repercussions of osteoporosis. You can't just go out and rent a new skeleton!

✓ Older adults and childbearing women can significantly improve bladder control by performing just 5 minutes of pelvic floor muscle exercises three times daily, according to the U.S. National Institute of Diabetes, Digestive, and Kidney Diseases.

✓ People who work out consistently often have other healthy lifestyle practices. They're less likely to indulge in smoking, excessive drinking, or overeating. There's a phenomenal domino effect; if you start an exercise program, you're more likely to choose more nutritious foods. It just makes sense!

✓ The body will be less prone to disease and illness. Two of the top killers—heart disease and cancer—can be reduced by up to 50 percent or more with positive lifestyle changes, including exercise. With increased circulation and oxygenation of the entire body, toxins and waste are eliminated more efficiently and nutrients are transported to areas they are needed. Exercise also prevents the build-up of fat and cholesterol in the arteries and decreases the chance of blood clots.

✓ In February 2005, the *Journal of Neurology* reported 60 percent less risk of Parkinson's for those participating in regular physical activity in early adult life. Parkinson's is a chronic, degenerative disease of the central nervous system that afflicts more than 1.5 million people in North America. People with Parkinson's have a full-blown deficiency in a neurotransmitter called dopamine, which makes you feel alert and gives you emotional drive. Sam Graci, in *The Path to Phenomenal Health*, recommends activities like resistance training, Pilates, martial arts, and mountain biking to increase your dopamine levels.

> **Health Miracle**
>
> The *Journal of the American Medical Association*, published in 2005, reported that breast cancer risk is lowered by about 50 percent in exercisers.

The Fitness Prescription

The majority of obesity experts agree that the dramatic increase in obesity in U.S. society [over] the last few decades is not attributable to genetics.
   —Len Kravitz, Ph.D.

You might be saying, "But I play tennis all summer," or "I play hockey on the weekends, isn't that enough?" It's great that you are taking some action, but most sports follow a season, leaving you with no activity during the rest of the year. Also, you must take into consideration whether you will be able to participate in your sport for a lifetime. And, finally, most sports do not cover all the bases when it comes to your fitness.

There is a basic exercise prescription you should follow to maintain optimal health throughout the stages of your life. This prescription includes a few doses of aerobic activity, a drop or two of strength training, and a stretch every day to keep the doctor away. This prescription can be done forever.

Aerobic Activity

Aerobic exercise helps the heart pump more blood to the brain, along with the rest of the body. More blood means more oxygen, and thus better nourished brain cells.
   —Dr. John Ratey

Coronary artery disease (CAD) is a major problem for many countries in the world. In fact, it is the leading cause of death in developed countries. When your arteries become damaged, they no longer allow blood to flow properly to and from the heart. The heart muscle literally starves.

Aerobic activity, also known as cardiovascular activity, increases your heart rate and makes you breathe a little harder. When you are aerobically fit, you are able to walk for extended periods of time, catch a bus, climb stairs easily, and run quickly for short distances with a fast recovery (i.e., the heart rate returns to normal within minutes of exercise cessation).

Arteries tend to stiffen with age. In a 2002 study Dr. Kerrie Moreau showed a 50 percent improvement in elasticity of arteries in postmenopausal overweight and inactive women after a 13-week walking program combined with the usual hormone-replacement therapy. The women in the study walked five days per week for 40 minutes at a moderate pace.

Talk Test: How Hard Are You Working?

Light activity: Normal conversation is possible.

Moderate activity: Talking becomes difficult and you speak in fragments, with breaths in-between.

Intense activity: Talking is impossible.

Look around any gym and you will see that most people are engaged in light activity for their whole exercise program! We once saw a woman stop pedaling her exercise bike for over 10 minutes of her 20-minute ride while she talked on her cell phone. When her friend arrived and asked her how long she had been riding, she proclaimed that she had been "going hard for more than 20 minutes!"

Vary your aerobic activities to avoid overuse injuries. Jogging or running is a great cardiovascular activity, but it can cause joint damage if done daily for great lengths of time. Ask any full-time aerobic instructor about overuse injuries and we're sure he or she will tell you about the importance of moderation and variety.

Dr. Andrew Weil, founder and director of the University of Arizona's Program for Integrative Medicine, recommends that you aim to get into the moderate range for about 30 minutes most days of the week to experience the release of the feel-good hormones and to promote good blood flow. You also need to get your heart rate into the intense range a few times per week. Dr. Mehmet Oz and Dr. Michael Roizen recommend that you elevate your heart rate to about 80 percent of your age-adjusted maximum (calculation to determine your age-adjusted maximum: 220 – your age) for about 20 minutes three times per week. It has been shown that the pituitary gland in your brain unleashes human growth hormone (HGH) when you work in the higher-intensity ranges of aerobic exercise. Researchers have called HGH the "fountain of youth" hormone. It's known to help burn belly fat and stimulate muscle growth. Levels of this hormone naturally decrease as you age, but a sedentary lifestyle will speed up this decline.

> *Visit www.caloriesperhour.com to help you calculate caloric expenditure.*

Health Miracle

Aerobic exercise can improve cardiovascular fitness, even after 30 years of inactivity. A study by McGuire et al. revealed a 100 percent reversal of age-related declines in aerobic power in midlife men after only six months of endurance training!

Strength Training

Exercise is a high-yield investment opportunity that generates both short- and long-term measurable results.
   —Rod Macdonald, Vice President, Canadian Association
   of Fitness Professionals

The best way to maintain or promote muscle strength and bone density is by weight training or resistance training. Anyone, at any age, can benefit from resistance training. The more muscle tissue you have, the better your metabolic furnace! Exercise can decrease the loss of muscle mass, strength, and power as you age. This becomes very important when you consider that an inactive 70-year-old may have lost an estimated 50 percent of his or her strength, an obvious liability in caring for the home and garden! With muscle loss comes a drop in resting metabolic rate (by about 2–3 percent for each decade). This can be minimized with a regular resistance-training program.

Muscles and bones shrink with age, so it is important to combine aerobic work with some resistance training. Even as little as once a week is good for maintenance and joint protection, but twice a week can actually bolster strength, improve posture, and increase bone density, all important for an active older adult lifestyle. Bone is constantly being reformed in response to demands and stresses. Resistance exercise is a positive way to stimulate new bone formation.

Many people neglect this area of fitness. Most start a fitness program with weight loss in mind and mistakenly think that the fastest way to this goal is aerobic exercise. What they don't realize is that aerobic training, partnered with resistance training and a healthy nutrition plan, will ensure the fastest results in the best possible manner for your health. Aerobic activity and dieting alone can lead to accelerated muscle wasting and lowered metabolism. The result is even more weight gain when the participant "falls off the wagon." By combining aerobic training with strength training, you will burn more calories, preserve functional muscle tissue, and keep your metabolism elevated. This is the fastest way to get the results you want and the only way to change the shape of your body instead of just becoming a smaller version of the old you!

Results from a good resistance-training program can be felt quickly. In just a matter of weeks, you will notice that you are able to lift heavier weights with more confidence. This benefit transfers directly to your daily life when you open stiff doors, get in and out of your vehicle, carry your grocery bags, lift your children or grandchildren, and move your furniture around.

Many people are scared to go to the weight room if they are self-conscious and think everyone will be looking at them. Don't worry—all the beautiful people in the gym are too busy looking at themselves! The only time they might notice you is if you get between them and the mirror.

There are several options for resistance training. You can use your own body weight and simple, inexpensive pieces of equipment like Bosu balls, stability balls, and resistance bands. Another form of exercise that is very popular for its posture, strength, and flexibility benefits is Pilates. Or you can use a home gym that allows you to do several exercises with one large piece of equipment. Machines are typically safe, yet they are not as demanding as free weights and barbells. So, if you are looking to take your weight training to the next level, you may want to invest in a weight bench and an assortment of dumbbells. In our next chapter, "The Miracle of Health Workout," we have designed a program that encompasses all your training needs. You can get visual depictions of numerous exercises and pieces of equipment at our Web site: www.FitSpeakers.com.

If you are unfamiliar with resistance training, don't be scared to ask for help from a certified personal trainer. A certified trainer can teach you the correct breathing techniques, posture, and form necessary to get the most from your program and avoid injury.

Deb's Story

Last year I rejoined my health club and got connected up with a personal trainer that I clicked with and he made a big improvement in my life. I dropped double digits in body fat and the scale confirmed it as well. My attitude and my health improved, including getting off of insulin injections! When I started with my trainer, I told him that I could not run with my bad knees (two surgeries from skiing) and my bad back. Months later, after a strength training and aerobic program, he had me running a couple of laps around the track at the health club and on the following Mother's Day, I ran my first 3-mile race with him. I ran the entire distance and have since completed four more races this year with another three scheduled.

Health Miracle

Even just one session of 30 minutes of weight training/weight-bearing exercise per week can maintain muscle strength and bone density. You could split this up into two 15-minute sessions, or three 10-minute sessions per week.

Flexibility and Balance Training

Notice that the stiffest tree is most easily cracked, while the bamboo or willow survives by bending with the wind.
—Bruce Lee, martial arts legend

If you are a dog owner, you know exactly what your dog does every morning when it gets up. Yes, that's right—it stretches with wanton abandonment and complete enjoyment. It is not embarrassed or uncomfortable with the thought that someone might be watching. And it didn't go to university or take a fitness certification! Have you ever thought it might be a good idea to get down on all fours and stretch with your dog?

Animals seem to know instinctively that stretching feels good. In fact, it does much more than feel good. It keeps muscles supple and joints lubricated. This can eradicate many of the common aches and pains associated with stiffness and a sedentary lifestyle.

Yoga is an excellent practice as the *asanas*, or postures, stretch all of the major muscles. Yoga classes also include balance poses, which will increase your stability. If you are not interested in a formal yoga practice, it is easy enough to learn some basic stretches that you can perform anywhere, and many devices are available in most gyms or fitness stores for restoring and improving balance. Items like stability balls, Bosu balls, and balance boards all work balance and are relatively inexpensive for home use.

Tai chi is an excellent activity for balance. It comprises gentle, graceful movements done in sequence. It is referred to as a "soft" martial art, one that is especially enjoyed by active, older adults.

Health Miracle

Research shows that elderly tai chi participants are less likely to fall and less likely to incur injuries if they do fall.

Successful Weight Loss

Walking is the best possible exercise. Habituate yourself to walk very far.
—Thomas Jefferson, third president of the United States

The U.S. National Weight Control Registry (www.nwcr.ws) is a database of men and women who have lost 60 pounds or more and maintained this weight loss for five or more years. There are several similarities among the most successful losers of body weight:

1. They are all physically active. On average, they accumulate 250 minutes per week of moderate-intensity exercise.

2. They all monitor how much food they eat, eating a wide variety of foods, but paying close attention to how much fat is in their diet.

3. Most of them maintain some type of weight-change chart.

4. Most of them weigh themselves at least once per week.

5. They all eat a healthy breakfast and are very consistent in their exercise patterns.

6. Of all the thousands of successful weight-loss participants in this registry, walking was the most common choice of aerobic activity! Walking is the safest, most natural form of light aerobic activity.

> *Go to www.shapeup.org for more information about the 10,000 steps per day program.*

Health Miracle

Blood-starved tissue in the heart will send out signals for new blood supplies to develop. Your body can actually build new blood vessels to support the damaged ones. This is called a collateral blood supply. You can increase collateral blood supplies by exercising!

Health Miracle Activities

1. Do you engage in some form of resistance training, aerobic activity, and flexibility on a weekly basis? Which area(s) need(s) the most attention?

_____

2. What is one strategy from this chapter you will implement today?

_____

3. Who else in your life will benefit if you made a positive change?

_____

4. Close your eyes, take a few deep breaths, then think of your new exercise strategy. Now picture yourself taking the action step. Smile to yourself and nod as you see yourself reaping the benefits. Fast-forward one year and imagine the results.

Chapter 7

If only it were as easy to exercise as it is to eat!
—Kary and Uche Odiatu

The Miracle of Health Exercise Plan

Strength does not come from winning. Your struggles develop your strength. When you go through hardship and decide not to surrender, that is strength.
   —Arnold Schwarzenegger

The exercise recommendations in this chapter were designed with busy people in mind! Time is precious and we have created the ultimate plan to ensure that you reap all the benefits of fitness in the shortest amount of time possible. We have combined circuits of resistance exercises with cardiovascular intervals—you will be moving! By keeping your heart rate up, these Fit Formulas will ensure that you achieve cardiovascular, flexibility, fat-burning, and strength benefits in the same workout.

Physiologically speaking, one of the keys to success with training is *variety*. Your body is incredibly adaptable. One of the most frustrating things about exercise is the dreaded plateau. You make some significant changes in your life, you experience some results, and you get stuck in the rut of doing the same exercises, the same cardio, every time you hit the gym. Eventually your body stops changing. You stop losing fat and inches and your strength gains stall. Boredom and frustration soon set in, leading to a lack of motivation—and we all know what happens next. That comfortable couch, tasty pizza, and yummy ice cream start looking very appealing.

Variety

Variety is key! To stimulate all of your body's 640 muscles and allow for maximal improvements in strength and endurance, you need to vary weight, repetitions, and exercises. There are several ways you can aim for variety in your workouts:

- Try the same exercise with different equipment. A chest exercise can be performed as a machine chest press, a push-up from your knees, a push-up from your toes, a dumbbell incline press on a bench, a straight bar press on a flat bench, a dumbbell press on a ball, etc.

- Try using different intensities. One week you may aim for 8–10 repetitions, the next week you may aim for 10–12 reps, and the following week you might aim for 12–15 reps. Lift heavier weights in the lower repetition ranges to encourage strength gains. Lift less weight with higher numbers of repetitions to increase strength and emphasize the endurance of muscle fibers. You can gauge the amount of weight you should lift by the rep ranges. If you are unable to reach the lower end of the repetition range (i.e., you can perform only 7 reps and the prescription was 8–10 reps), then you are using too much weight. If you could easily do more than the prescribed repetition range, you need a heavier weight.

- Use different pieces of cardio equipment like a stepper, an elliptical, a treadmill, or a stationary bike.

- Try new and different classes (such as yoga, Pilates, cardio kickbox, etc.) throughout the year.

- Try new instructors. Each one brings different teaching styles and talents to his or her programs. There are *boot camp*-style instructors with little patience for slackers. There are also supportive and encouraging instructors who are great if you are a newbie.

- Try a new personal trainer, and interview your trainer before you make a commitment. Trainers differ greatly in their strengths, personalities, and experience levels. Many specialize in certain areas: older adults, sport-specific training, children's fitness, and transformation or weight loss.

Time

We know that most people feel they have a different amount of time they can commit to exercise, and we recognize that there are times in your life when you will be able to perform only resistance training once per week. This is why we have created three different Fit Formulas. You can choose the one that works best for your schedule, or you can rotate through the Fit Formulas every few weeks to provide extra stimulation and variety for your workouts.

Fit Formula One is a total-body workout that will give you benefits in just two workouts per week. If you have a week where you can work out only once, then this is the formula to use since it will challenge all of your muscles and maintain your current strength. Fit Formula Two increases the intensity of the program by instructing you to perform fewer repetitions but using more weight. Fit Formula Two can be done two or three times per week. Fit Formula Three includes three separate workouts with a higher intensity. Ideally, you would commit to three workouts per week with Fit Formula Three.

Our formulas allow you to choose your own exercises. Just plug them into the formula and get started. We have created a huge resource of exercises on our Web site that can be done at the gym or at home. There are exercises for all ranges of ability, from beginner to advanced. Visit our Web site at www.FitSpeakers.com to view several pictures of various forms of cardiovascular activity and a wide variety of resistance exercises to spice up your workout routine. You can also print out the Fit Formulas so that you will not have to carry the book into the gym!

At the end of your workouts, we have suggested a brief cooldown period of stretching. Flexibility gains are best made when the body is warm, so following your workout is the best time to increase your flexibility. Use your own stretches, or visit our Web site for some quick yoga/stretching sequences to round out your workout. Remember to move slowly into your stretches. You should feel some tension as you relax into the stretch, but not pain. Hold your stretches for a minimum of 10 seconds. The longer you are able to stay in the stretch, the more you will increase your flexibility for the part of the body you are stretching. Breathe deeply and slowly as you ease deeper into the stretch. An inability to breathe will indicate that you need to ease up your stretch.

Just by using these formulas you will experience great benefits to your health. On days that you are not using the Fit Formulas, you should still aim for about 30–60 minutes of physical activity done at a moderate intensity. Government health agencies in Canada and the U.S. recommend most days of the week, which means that minimally you should aim to be active at least five of the seven days. So, if you are doing Fit Formula One or Fit Formula Two, you should aim for about 30 minutes of physical activity on at least three other days of your week. If you are using Fit Formula Three, you only need to do some form of aerobic activity like vigorous walking, dancing, or your favorite group class on the other two days!

The United States Department of Health and Human Services reports that greater health benefits are gained when exercise is done at greater intensity and for longer duration. However, they also caution against excessive amounts of exercise, which can increase the risk of injury. Most of us need not worry about this because less than 10 percent of North Americans regularly perform exercise that includes aerobic conditioning, resistance training, and flexibility.

Health Miracle

The American College of Sports Medicine issued a statement in 2005 that substantial health benefits will come with regular, moderate-intensity physical activity (a brisk 2-mile walk that takes about 30 minutes, for example) five days per week.

Caution

If you have been sedentary, you need to get medical clearance before you begin any new program. And if you have any pre-existing medical conditions like heart disease, diabetes, or obesity, you must work together with your medical professional and a certified trainer to ensure a safe transition to an active lifestyle. You should aim to work toward one 10-minute session of physical activity in the beginning. Gradually increase this every few days and know that it is still beneficial to perform small increments of physical activity throughout your day. This will also keep your resolve strong.

Start with basic movements like walking, stretching, and some body-weight exercises (push-ups against a wall, squats with the aid of a chair, and abdominal exercises) followed by gentle stretching.

Once you are able to participate in physical activity for at least 30 consecutive minutes, you can start with Fit Formula One, working at your own pace. It is extremely important to get the help of a certified trainer if you are new to resistance training. You need to learn proper technique and breathing. You will also need to learn how to safely use equipment, whether it is in your own home or a gym.

> *There is a bright side to being a beginner! When you are new to a sport or activity, you will actually burn more calories per hour during that activity than someone who is proficient at it. In the beginning, you need to expend a lot of effort and make more attempts to achieve the desired results. For example, a beginner at golf will have to take many more strokes than a professional, so he or she will burn more calories.*

If you are healthy (as deemed by your medical professional), and you are familiar with the basics of resistance training, then you are ready to get started. Lace up your shoes and try Fit Formula One!

Health Miracle

Even a 5–10 percent modest weight loss of initial body weight for overweight women can significantly lower blood pressure.

Know Your Numbers

Take care of your body. It's the only place you have to live.
—Jim Rohn, author and business philosopher

Have your medical doctor perform the following tests before you start your exercise program: blood pressure test, cholesterol test, homocysteine, c-reactive protein, and blood sugar levels. Your doctor may give you "normal" values for the tests (i.e., Your doctor will tell you that your blood pressure is "normal" at 120 over 80, yet this is the bottom number for high blood pressure!), but you want to ask for the "ideal" values so that you can focus your efforts on ideal health. Remember that over 60 percent of the North American population is out of shape, so why be a part of the norm? Re-evaluate in six months and see how quickly your body responds!

Michelle's Story

You might call me a "late bloomer" when it comes to dancing. I didn't start formal dance training until I was 18 years old, so this impacted my confidence and self-esteem when it came to networking with other dancers or auditioning for parts. By the age of 26 I thought that I was done with my dancing. . . . I had surgery to repair a torn ACL ligament and this took me away from my passion for close to a year.

During the recovery months I could not help but notice the growing interest in dancing that seemed to be taking over the networks. Shows like "Dancing with the Stars" and "So You Think You Can Dance" had me glued to the TV. Something was burning inside me. I wanted to prove that I was a GOOD dancer. You see, I had never given my passion 100 percent. I was 5 feet 6 inches and close to 150 pounds—not ideal for a dancer who takes herself seriously!

My fitness mentors, Kary and Uche Odiatu, said they would help me prepare for the Canadian auditions of "So You Think You Can Dance." They gave me the Miracle of Health Exercise Plan to follow and instead of a diet, they helped me slowly switch my snacks and meals to healthier choices and smaller portions. I never had to count calories, and I even enjoyed the occasional glass of wine.

The Fit Formulas never took more than one hour (two to three times per week). They flew by because the cardio and weight lifting were split up. I HAD NEVER EXPERIENCED SO MUCH SWEAT BEFORE! The results were immediate. One week after starting, my energy was higher and my motivation was stronger. Six months later I had lost 17 pounds and my body looked toned for the first time since high school! I didn't even know that I had that much body fat to lose!

My audition is coming up soon, but I am more excited about my newfound confidence with dancing and my body. I perform with much more energy because I feel good inside and out. This has had such a domino effect on my entire life. And now I have finally proven that I am a GREAT dancer to the most important person—myself!

Steps to Exercise Success

The *Journal of Sports Medicine and Physical Fitness* reported that over half of all men and 65 percent of women who begin a regular exercise and nutrition program drop out within three months. To avoid being a statistic, you can bolster yourself by trying the following:

- Get your physician's approval before starting any physical fitness program.

- Make a public statement to key people in your life about your goals for the future. In the beginning, you may not be comfortable sharing with anyone. That's okay! It all depends on the people you have in your life. Share with people who will support you, not criticize or ridicule you. A new goal is like a baby, who needs support and nurturing. Our last chapter will help you develop goals that will inspire your fitness journey!

- Keep an exercise log and record your efforts and improvements. This can be highly motivating and excellent for reviewing your progress and setting new goals. You can include your physiological numbers (blood pressure, etc.), the increases in strength as reflected by the weight you can lift or an increase in reps for a given weight, and you may include weight, inches, or body composition results. Body composition must be done by a fitness professional, who will calculate your body fat percentage by using skin-fold measurements from a caliper and plugging these measurements into equations with some girth measurements.

- Take "before" pictures of yourself from all four sides before you begin your plan of action. Every month take more pictures. Take the pictures wearing the same clothing in the same room. Have the photographer stand the same distance from you each time, with the same lighting. Your mind will often lag behind your progress—you probably know someone who made some major changes, yet he or she still feels fat. By actually looking at a picture, you can start to make the psychological adjustment to your new body.

- Give yourself some variety by walking, hiking, running, cycling, or even indoor rock climbing to put some spice into your training program. Cross-training prevents overuse injuries and boredom and provides for overall development. The key is to put an increased demand on your heart and lungs and use the large muscle groups of the body in a variety of ways.

- Choose an event to train for such as a local charity walk, a 3-mile race, a half-marathon, an office challenge, a bike race, a triathalon, a canoe trip, a mountain climb, etc.

- Choose a time to exercise and stick to it, so you can have a scheduled routine. By making it a "must" instead of a "should," you feel more committed to do what you say. In the beginning of your program, it's very important to honor your commitment. Missing just one session can lead to many more missed workouts. As you become more committed to your exercise routine, you will be able to miss a workout here and there without falling off the wagon for an extended period.

- Make a commitment to celebrate your victory over complacency every time you work out. People have a tendency to celebrate only large goals or milestones, like losing 20 pounds or winning a competition. The human psyche loves reinforcement. Without rewards along the way, it's very easy to become disillusioned and discouraged.

- Relax and have some patience. We often get e-mails and calls from new exercisers asking us when they will see results. We ask them how long they have been physically active and the reply is usually "A few weeks." Abs and buns of steel don't magically appear overnight. You have to remember how many years your body went without physical activity or good nutrition, so how can you expect to turn it around in a few weeks? Try focusing on how you are feeling and the sense of accomplishment that comes from maintaining your resolve instead of checking your stomach in the mirror every morning. It's like waiting for the kettle to boil—it can take forever if you sit and stare at it!

- Be a lifelong student. Learn about exercise (techniques and principles) and nutrition. Get a subscription to an exercise magazine, such as *Muscle and Fitness, Muscle and Fitness Hers, Men's Health, Fit Parent Magazine, Men's Fitness, Oxygen, Shape,* or *Alive.* There are also many videos and books available.

• Observe and talk to others who have made transformations and maintained them. Their testimonies will inspire you and give you confidence that it can be done.

• Work out with a partner and share the experience. You can enjoy the physical benefits together and strengthen the bond of your relationship. You will be less likely to skip workouts if someone else is depending on you to be there.

• Get certified! Many organizations offer weekend courses in personal training. There will be people of all shapes, sizes, and experience levels, so don't feel intimidated. You don't have to become a personal trainer, but why not learn the proper techniques and exercises for yourself?

Resistance Training Basics

Start with light resistance: Leave your ego in the locker-room! Gain mastery over the movement before attempting a heavier weight and you will enjoy a lifetime of weight training.

Breathing: Do not hold your breath while resistance training. This can be dangerous and is an indication that the load may be too heavy for you. Maintain a steady breathing pattern throughout the exercise. A certified trainer can help you learn how to exhale while you are doing the most work, which is the most effective way to breathe during weight training.

Don't lock your elbows and knees: Your knee and elbow joints should be soft, or slightly flexed (bent); avoid locking these joints.

Aim for a slow and steady movement speed during exercises: This has been proven to fire more muscle fibers and is much safer.

Engage your core: Pull in your abdominal muscles (belly button to spine), which will build up the strength of your midsection and will ensure good posture throughout your exercises.

Train within the rep range: If the rep range is 8–10, choose a weight that you can lift eight times, but not more than 10.

Hire a trainer: If you have any doubts or concerns about your exercise technique, this will be one of the best investments you will make!

Fit Formula One

> ### How to Find a Certified Trainer or Course in Your Area
> *American Council on Exercise:*
> *www.acefitness.org*
> *Canadian Fitness Professionals:*
> *www.canfitpro.com*
> *Holistic health care provider Paul Chek's Web site:*
> *www.chekinstitute.com*
> *Find a C.H.E.K. certified trainer:* ww.ideafit.com
> *National Strength and Conditioning Association:*
> *www.nsca-lift.org*

This formula is a twice weekly full-body workout, which is great if you have a week where your time for exercise is limited. At least you will get a full-body workout if you complete the formula once in your week. In this workout, you are aiming for 12–15 repetitions (reps) of each exercise. Use enough resistance so that it is almost impossible to perform more than 15 reps. Then you'll know you have done the job! Move from one exercise to the next with minimal rest in-between. A little rest is needed because you are working different muscle groups.

Next, head straight to your choice for cardiovascular activity, such as treadmill walking. Start at a moderate intensity for 2 minutes (you can still talk, but need to breathe deeper and start to break a light sweat), then increase the intensity by speeding up the pace or raising the incline of the treadmill so that you have to concentrate to perform the activity (talking should be difficult). For some of you, this would be a run or a jog on the treadmill; for others, a fast walk might be all you need (this is usually the case if you have been sedentary). When you first start these formulas, you will have to build up your ability to perform high-intensity intervals. It may take a few weeks before you can maintain a high intensity for 1 minute.

See how long you can maintain this intensity in the beginning and add to your time each workout. It's okay if you can handle only

10 seconds of high intensity—it will be only a matter of weeks until your endurance improves!

After your burst of high-intensity cardio, go back to 2 minutes of moderate-intensity cardio, then one more burst of high-intensity cardio. Now you are ready to repeat the repetition exercises you just did (or you may choose a new exercise, but work the same muscles). Since your muscles are warmed up at this point, you may want to aim for the lower end of the rep range this time (i.e., 12 reps). This would mean using a slightly heavier resistance, or performing the exercise more slowly. Follow this set of reps with another round of cardio and then continue to repeat the process for each muscle group as listed in Fit Formula One Workout. Note that once you get to shoulders and abs, the cardio interval is done only once.

Fit Formula One Workout

5-minutes of low-intensity warm-up on your choice of aerobic equipment

Leg, chest, back (aim for 15 reps each)

Perform one exercise for each, one after the other, with little or no rest between muscle groups.

2 minutes of moderate-intensity cardio, 1 minute of intense cardio

Perform this twice.

Leg, chest, back (aim for 12 reps each)

Perform the same exercise for each, or choose a different exercise, with little or no rest between muscle groups.

2 minutes of moderate-intensity cardio, 1 minute of intense cardio

Perform this twice.

Shoulders, abs (aim for 15 reps each)

Perform one exercise for each, with little or no rest between muscle groups.

2 minutes of moderate-intensity cardio, 1 minute of intense cardio

Perform this twice.

Shoulders, abs (aim for 12 reps each)

Perform the same exercise for each, or choose a different exercise, with little or no rest between muscle groups.

2 minutes of moderate-intensity cardio, 1 minute of intense cardio

Perform once.

Biceps, triceps (aim for 15 reps each)

Perform one exercise for each, with little or no rest between muscle
   groups.
2 minutes of moderate cardio, 1 minute of intense cardio
Perform once.
Biceps, triceps (aim for 12 reps each)
Perform the same exercise for each, or choose a different exercise,
   with little or no rest between muscle groups.
5–10 minutes of a cool-down series of stretches

Fit Formula Two

This formula is broken into two separate workouts: Workout #1 (back,
chest, abdominals, and calves) and Workout #2 (legs, shoulders, biceps,
and triceps). In this formula you are aiming for 10–12 repetitions for
each exercise. You can perform each workout once during the week to
complete a full body workout by the end of the week. We recommend
at least one or two days between workouts. Or you can increase your
strength and tone even more by following a three-workout-per-week
schedule by alternating workouts: Workout #1 on Monday, active living on Tuesday, Workout #2 on Wednesday, active living on Thursday,
Workout #1 on Friday, rest days on Saturday and Sunday. The following week would start with Workout #2 on Monday.

Fit Formula Two, Workout #1: Back, Chest, Calves, and Abs
5 minutes of low-intensity warm-up on cardiovascular equipment
Back, chest (aim for 12 reps each)
Perform first exercise for each, then take 30 seconds of rest.
Back, chest (aim for 10 reps each)
Repeat the first exercise with more resistance or slower reps.
2 minutes of moderate cardio, 1 minute of intense cardio
Perform twice.
Back, chest (aim for 10 reps each)
Perform a second exercise for each.
2 minutes of moderate cardio, 1 minute of intense cardio
Perform twice.
Calves, abs (aim for 12 reps each)
Perform first exercise for each, then take 30 seconds of rest.
Calves, abs (aim for 10 reps each)

Repeat the first exercise with more resistance or slower reps.

2 minutes of moderate cardio, 30 seconds of intense cardio

Perform twice.

Calves, abs (aim for 10 reps each)

Perform a second exercise for each.

2 minutes of moderate cardio, 30 seconds of intense cardio

Perform twice.

5–10 minutes of a cool-down series of stretches

Fit Formula Two, Workout #2: Legs, Shoulders, Biceps, and Triceps

5 minutes of low-intensity warm-up on cardiovascular equipment

Legs, shoulders (aim for 12 reps each)

Perform one exercise for each, then take 30 seconds of rest.

Legs, shoulders (aim for 10 reps each)

Repeat the first exercise with more resistance or slower reps.

2 minutes of moderate cardio, 1 minute of intense cardio

Perform twice.

Legs, shoulders (aim for 10 reps each)

Perform a second exercise for each.

2 minutes of moderate cardio, 1 minute of intense cardio

Perform twice.

Biceps, triceps (aim for 12 reps each)

Perform one exercise for each, then take 30 seconds of rest.

Biceps, triceps (aim for 10 reps each)

Repeat the first exercise with more resistance or slower reps.

2 minutes of moderate cardio, 30 seconds of intense cardio

Perform twice.

Biceps, triceps (aim for 10 reps each)

Perform a second exercise for each.

2 minutes of moderate cardio, 30 seconds of intense cardio

Perform twice.

5–10 minutes of a cool-down series of stretches

Fit Formula Three

In this formula the entire body is broken into three separate workouts. Aim for 8–10 repetitions for each exercise. Since you are aiming for three sets of each exercise and a low rep range, more recovery time is needed and each body part is trained only once per week. With the lower rep range the cardio between exercises will be only a moderate cardio. You will still get the fat-burning benefits, but it will allow your body a chance to recover for the next set.

Fit Formula Three, Workout #1: Back, Chest

5 minutes of low-intensity warm-up on cardio equipment
Back, chest (aim for 10 reps)
Perform one exercise for each.
3 minutes of moderate-intensity cardio
Back, chest (aim for 8 reps)
Repeat the first exercise with more resistance or slower reps.
3 minutes of moderate-intensity cardio
Back, chest (aim for 8 reps)
Repeat the first exercise; it should be tough to do the 8 reps.
3 minutes of moderate-intensity cardio
Back, chest (aim for 10 reps)
Perform a second exercise for each.
3 minutes of moderate-intensity cardio
Back, chest (aim for 8 reps)
Repeat the second exercise with more resistance or slower reps.
3 minutes of moderate-intensity cardio
Back, chest (aim for 8 reps)
Repeat the second exercise; it should be tough to do the 8 reps.
10 minutes of moderate-intensity cardio to finish
5–10 minutes of a cool-down series of stretches

Fit Formula Three, Workout #2: Legs, Abs

5 minutes of low-intensity warm-up on cardio equipment
Legs, abs (aim for 10 reps)
Perform one exercise for each.
3 minutes of moderate-intensity cardio
Legs, abs (aim for 8 reps)
Repeat the first exercise with more resistance or slower reps.
3 minutes of moderate-intensity cardio
Legs, abs (aim for 8 reps)
Repeat the first exercise; it should be tough to do the 8 reps.
3 minutes of moderate-intensity cardio
Legs, abs (aim for 10 reps)

Perform a second exercise for each.

3 minutes of moderate-intensity cardio

Legs, abs (aim for 8 reps)

Repeat the second exercise with more resistance or slower reps.

3 minutes of moderate-intensity cardio

Legs, abs (aim for 8 reps)

Repeat the second exercise; it should be tough to do the 8 reps.

10 minutes of moderate-intensity cardio to finish

5–10 minutes of a cool-down series of stretches

Fit Formula Three, Workout #3: Shoulders, Biceps, Triceps

5 minutes of low-intensity warm-up on cardio equipment

Shoulders, biceps, triceps (aim for 10 reps)

Perform one exercise for each.

3 minutes of moderate-intensity cardio

Shoulders, biceps, triceps (aim for 8 reps)

Repeat the first exercise with more resistance or slower reps.

3 minutes of moderate-intensity cardio

Shoulders, biceps, triceps (aim for 8 reps)

Repeat the first exercise; it should be tough to do the 8 reps.

3 minutes of moderate-intensity cardio

Shoulders, biceps, triceps (aim for 10 reps)

Perform a second exercise for each.

3 minutes of moderate-intensity cardio

Shoulders, biceps, triceps (aim for 8 reps)

Repeat the second exercise with more resistance or slower reps.

3 minutes of moderate-intensity cardio

Shoulders, biceps, triceps (aim for 8 reps)

Repeat the second exercise; it should be tough to do the 8 reps.

10 minutes of moderate-intensity cardio to finish

5–10 minutes of a cool-down series of stretches

Chapter 8

Up to a point a man's life is shaped by environment, heredity, and movements and changes in the world about him. Then there comes a time when it lies within his grasp to shape the clay of his life into the sort of thing he wishes to be. Only the weak blame parents, their race, their times, lack of good fortune, or the quirks of fate.
—Louis L'Amour

No Excuses!

Physical fitness is the basis for all other forms of excellence.
    —John F. Kennedy

When it comes to weight loss and better health you can either make *excuses* or get *results*. We have heard every excuse on the planet as to why someone can't exercise, and we have also met people who can blow every excuse you have out of the water! Take our friend, Sean Stephenson (www.seanstephenson.com), for example. Sean was born with a life-threatening disease called osteogenesis imperfecta (brittle-bone disease). When he was born, he had so many fractures that the doctors gave him a slim chance of living. He did live, and he has survived hundreds of fractures to become a motivational force. Sean never was able to walk due to deformities from so many breaks and is confined to a wheelchair, but he still hired a personal trainer to strengthen his body and started eating a healthy diet, and was rewarded with more confidence and fewer fractures. Sean inspires us on a daily basis to say: *No excuses!*

Health Miracle

Rev up your immune system with moderate exercise. People who exercise catch fewer colds.

Take Responsibility

All blame is a waste of time. No matter how much fault you find with another, and regardless of how much you blame him, it will not change you.
—Wayne Dyer, Ph.D.

We went to one of the great success gurus for help with this topic. Jack Canfield, in his book *The Success Principles*, tells of a formula that was given to him by a psychotherapist, Dr. Robert Resnick. The principle behind the formula is that you must take 100 percent responsibility for everything in your life. When you blame outside circumstances for all that has gone wrong in your life, you give up your own personal power. We agree. You can't change if you feel that outside forces like your spouse, children, coworkers, etc., are the cause of all your woes. His formula is: E + R = O (Event + Response = Outcome).

So, if you are not enjoying your current outcomes, then you can either blame the E (event) or change your R (response). If you make the first choice, you may find yourself experiencing the same outcome over and over. If everyone blamed someone or some outside event for their unwanted outcomes, we would not have any successful people on the planet!

By making the second choice, or changing our responses, we claim our power to act and think differently and when we try again, we may still fail, but eventually we will find the right response to have a successful outcome.

An example that demonstrates this concept came from a former client who was the mother of a young girl. The mother constantly repeated the phrase: "Ever since I had her, I have been overweight." She not only said this to us, she said this in front of her daughter. The implication of this statement was that the child (or the event of having a child) was responsible for the mother's excess weight. This has two negative consequences: first of all, the child feels blamed for the mother's weight gain, and second, the mother is not admitting that her lack of exercise and poor food choices are responsible for the excess weight.

She has given up the power to do something about her excess weight. If her assumption that having children makes you fat was correct, then every woman on the planet with children would be overweight. That's an absurd belief, but if you dig deep, most of the beliefs that hold you back from getting what you want are absurd.

Once the mother takes personal responsibility for her body, she will be able to change her responses and make new positive lifestyle changes to support her desire for weight loss. And this small adjustment opens the window for a health miracle to occur.

Health Miracle

Movement helps you feel rejuvenated. Experts in the field report that just 10–15 minutes of brisk walking may provide approximately 2 hours of elevated energy levels. After a long day at work, try some exercise before you return home to your family.

People Who Said "No Excuses"

Obstacles don't have to stop you.
If you run into a wall, don't turn around and give up.
Figure out a way to climb it, go through it, or work around it.
　　—Michael Jordan, NBA superstar

- Ted Turner was 24 when his father committed suicide. Ted went on to become the founder of CNN by parlaying his father's modest business into a huge media empire. He did not let a diagnosis of manic depression corral him into limitations. With almost 2 million acres of land, he is North America's largest individual landowner and has given billions to charity.

- Arnold Schwarzenegger immigrated to the U.S. in 1968. He barely spoke any English and had less than $20 in his pocket. Since then he has become a number-one box office actor and governor of California.

- Abraham Lincoln became president of the United States regardless of numerous election defeats, a history of personal bankruptcy, and many family tragedies.

- Joan Rivers survived near financial ruin and the tragic suicide of her husband only to have a great comeback in her sixties. She now has a successful jewelry line and has established herself as one of the great entertainers of all time.

• Dr. Wayne Dyer is one of the world's foremost inspirational gurus. He was raised in an orphanage after his father abandoned his family.

• Oprah Winfrey has become one of the most influential people in North America. She was raised in an abusive environment and had a stillborn baby during her teen years.

• Sam Walton, legendary founder of Wal-Mart, grew up during the Depression in a family divided by divorce.

• Louise Hay survived incest and physical abuse to become a best-selling author, lecturer, and publisher. She has helped millions of people with personal growth and self-healing.

Excuse Busters

EXCUSE: Exercise hurts!

REALITY: An audience member once told us that she had tried a resistance program and experienced pain in her muscles and knee joints. We politely asked if she had ever received proper instruction from a certified trainer and she replied "No." We then asked how long she had been on her program, to which she replied: "I never went back because it hurt so much." We explained that a certain amount of stiffness or soreness in muscle tissue was a completely normal response after attempting a new activity. That's why it's so important to start out slowly with low intensity. Your muscle fibers break down a little when you challenge them, which means you will experience some soreness or stiffness as your body repairs the tissue. This is how muscle adapts. Your amazing body grows stronger each time it does its special repair job. The next time you perform the same activity, your body will have adapted and will not be as sore unless you work harder by increasing the demand again.

Pain in the knee or any joint is a different matter. You should not experience pain in the actual joints. It could mean that you were doing an exercise with poor technique or with too much resistance. Start with a certified trainer who can ensure that you are following appropriate exercise guidelines. If the joint pain does not go away, you may need better footwear, or you may need to seek counsel from your health care practitioner to determine the cause of the pain. Ask your health care provider to recommend a physiotherapist or athletic therapist. There are risks inherent in trying anything new, so make sure that you are well equipped for your exercise, and enlist help in the beginning!

EXCUSE: I exercise, so I can eat whatever I want.

REALITY: To maximize the full benefits of exercise, you need foods high in nutrients. Nutritional deficiencies can occur if you exercise with a depleted body. Many people start an exercise program without making any nutritional changes, or they eat even more of the wrong foods because they think that the increase in activity justifies it. And then they wonder why they don't see weight-loss results. Too often, they quit their programs, chalking their weight problems up to genetics or a thyroid problem. The best plan includes regular exercise and changes to your diet, small steps taken over a long period of time. Like compound interest in a savings account, exponential growth occurs.

EXCUSE: I have to lose some body fat before I start resistance training.

REALITY: Resistance training is one of the best ways to help you lose fat. When you lift weights, you can significantly increase your metabolic rate (the rate at which your body burns calories). When you add more muscle fibers to your frame (or get more toned), your body requires more energy to maintain that muscle tone. Muscle tissue burns approximately 50 times more calories compared to fat. Both men and women receive benefits from building lean muscle mass. Aerobic exercise can get you into a fat-burning zone for a short period of time, but adding more muscle raises your thermostat for the long haul.

EXCUSE: I'm too tired to work out after a long day at the office.

REALITY: The hormones associated with physical activity will re-energize and revitalize you. Once you get yourself moving, you'll be glad you did—physically and psychologically! Believe us, there are days when we don't feel like going to the gym either. And there's the occasional time when we don't go. One thing is for sure: we don't regret going! Exercise gives you that second wind for the rest of your day.

EXCUSE: Being a woman, I'm afraid I'll get bulky if I lift weights.

REALITY: Did you know that fat takes up more space than muscle? In other words, losing fat and toning muscle means that even though you may weigh the same, your problem areas will be much smaller (think of your hips and thighs). You can change your shape dramatically by adding more muscle to your upper body while toning the lower body and burning fat, creating the appearance of a smaller waist and thighs.

Muscles do not show up overnight! It's a gradual process, and you are totally in control of how much muscle you develop. Once you are satisfied with your level of muscle tone, you can follow a maintenance program. Muscles will not keep growing unless they are constantly challenged with increasing weights or intensity. It's not as if one morning you will wake up with arms like Arnold Schwarzenegger's!

EXCUSE: You have to lift weights every day to strengthen muscle.

REALITY: Muscles are broken down during exercise. It is the *rest time* following the workout when the body repairs the muscle tissue, making it even stronger and bigger. If you are not giving your body enough rest/recovery/regrowth time, you won't experience gains in strength or size. The body part that has been trained requires about 48 hours to recover properly. There are many different ways to schedule your workouts in a week to maximize your training. There are many programs that will work: the key is to find something you enjoy and can implement into your life. Pick one to start, and then experiment with others and make your own choices. Again, this is where a personal trainer or your own research will be of value. The key is to start now!

EXCUSE: I have so much to do. I'll get started next week.

REALITY: Waiting for the perfect time is a no-win situation. Before you know it, weeks and then years have gone by. The consequences slowly sneak up on you. It's like a nagging toothache. The pain and anguish could have been avoided by early prevention. However, it's not always easy to do what we know we should do. In the beginning you will need to call upon your willpower to get you moving, even if it is only for 10 or 15 minutes. You will still be doing your body and mind some good! You have the power to make any time the right time.

EXCUSE: I don't like exercise.

REALITY: There is hope for you! There will be initial resistance, especially if you are sedentary and "hate" exercise. Just do it! Eventually you will feel uncomfortable if you don't! We told the story of Kary's sister, Laurie, in the beginning of the book. She hated exercise, but after a year of forcing herself to get to the gym, she finally came to the conclusion that exercise makes her a better person. She has more energy and feels better able to deal with her heavy workload and her family on the days she heads to the gym during her lunch hour.

EXCUSE: I feel guilty about not spending enough time with family or friends.

REALITY: When we ask our audiences for the reasons why they don't exercise, inevitably a woman will hold up her hand and say "Guilt." We are not trying to infer that men don't feel guilty about taking time for their interests outside of the home, but we have yet to hear this response from a man!

For all you men out there, try to understand that you may need to lovingly push your wife or female significant other out the door and reassure her that it's okay for her to take care of herself.

And for all the women out there who give, give, and give: You will eventually wear yourself out, and then you won't be able to nurture the important people in your life. Remember when we talked about balance and living in the present moment? Well, this goes for all areas of your life, even though it breaks your heart to leave the kids. Once you are out of the door, you have to focus on the task at hand and allow yourself to enjoy what you are doing. You will be home again soon enough!

We have interviewed many parents who manage to exercise, make time for each other, and spend quality time with their children. Here are some of their tips:

- Share duties with another family. Take turns looking after each other's children.

- Make the kids part of a fitness night out. Include activities they would like and that you would like (e.g., family skating, swimming, or bike riding).

- Join a facility that caters to all ages and provides programming for your children while you participate in your own activity.

- Join a facility that offers quality child care. A great workout can take less than an hour!

- Be a role model. Taking the time for your own health will set the standard for your children's future. Your children are watching your every move.

- Avoid using your children as an excuse for not having time to invest in your own health. Children pick up on these messages and take them to heart!

- See time with your children as an opportunity to try new activities or relearn activities you enjoyed when you were their age.

EXCUSE: I travel a lot—it's impossible to stay healthy on the road.

REALITY: Is it possible to stick to a health and fitness regimen when traveling? Of course! But it isn't easy. People are always a little intrigued when they discover that we maintain our fitness strategies when we travel. Most believe our commitment must just be super strong. Sure it's strong. But the truth is if we can do it, anyone can.

A vacation or business trip *can* include fitness and sound nutrition. A vacation is also a perfect opportunity to try some new activities; they may even last a lifetime, long after your tan wears off. The habit of training at a gym, rock climbing or going for evening walks could possibly be the greatest souvenir to bring home with you! Here are some tips for your next trip:

- **Affirm:** Declare daily the importance of staying true to your nutritional goals before you leave. Remind yourself of the hard work and effort you have put toward your fitness so far. Decide ahead that you will follow sound nutritional practices 80 percent of the time, so you will be able to enjoy the occasional indulgence. And commit to at least a walk every day.

- **Hydrate:** Drink plenty of water before you head out. A well-hydrated body is less prone to jet lag, water retention, and headaches. Don't forget to purchase bottled water after you pass through security at the airport: that shot glass of water you get from the flight attendant is barely enough to wet your whistle! If you are well hydrated, you will be less likely to make poor choices like pop or alcohol.

- **Pack snacks:** Some of the downsides of traveling include missed flights, long waits, delays, and expensive airport food. There are many tasty, healthy snacks that are easy to pack in a small cooler. We always travel with a supply of veggies, meal-replacement bars, rice cakes, fruit, hard-boiled eggs, and hummus wraps. These are food items that can be eaten anywhere: in a long lineup rescheduling a flight, waiting for the next flight in an airport lounge, or in a taxi on the way to your hotel. Bring some Ziploc bags along; if the security staff take away your ice pack, you can always fill up the Ziploc bag with ice at an airport restaurant.

- **Call ahead:** We always call ahead to book a refrigerator for our room. Sometimes there is a small charge for this. This charge is sometimes waived if you are using the fridge for medication, so bring along your fish oil supplements and tell the reception staff that you need the fridge for your medicine!

- **Hit the local supermarket:** One of your first destinations upon arrival should be a local grocery store where you can stock up on some food items for the hotel room. Excellent choices are multigrain bagels, hummus, apples, rice cakes, bananas, nuts, rye bread, tuna, and salmon. Buy the cans with the pull-off lids if you forget a can opener. Buy instant oatmeal to prepare in the room using hot water from the coffee maker or ask for a small electric kettle. This idea will save you from the late-night hotel vending-machine munchies. Plus, having a quick breakfast in your room means more time for sightseeing!

- **Exercise:** Try to book a hotel that has an on-site facility or a gym nearby. Even a half-hour workout done two or three times during the vacation will refresh you and help to maintain your current fitness level. We try to get in some physical activity as soon as we arrive at our destination. It's amazing how quickly you can get a second wind and recover from the jetlag!

EXCUSE: I'm too old to make any significant changes to my body.

REALITY: At about the age of 25, your muscle mass starts to deteriorate and your body-fat stores increase if you do not add resistance training, proper nutrition, and cardiovascular training to your life. With this decrease in muscle and increase in fat, we become fragile, weak, and prone to injury. Bill Phillips mentions in his book, *Body-for-Life*, a study from Tufts University in which a three-times-per-week weight-training program done with men ages 60–72 caused an increase in flexibility and strength of up to 200 percent. The best thing is that anyone can start weight training today and reap the rewards! Read on to learn some of these benefits in the next chapter, "Active Older Adult."

AND THE NUMBER-ONE EXCUSE: I don't have time.

REALITY: It is unbelievable that people in the Western world spend so much time watching television. Okay, we acknowledge there is some excellent programming on television. But the average house in North America has the TV switched on seven hours a day. The average person watches about 20 hours a week, with a large number watching as much as 35 hours a week. That is almost a full-time job! Maybe you could use 30 minutes of this time to get out for a walk or buy an exercise bike to place in front of your big screen TV!

It is definitely possible to make gains with short, intense workouts. There's no need for marathon sessions to enjoy the rewards of exercise. Even 15 minutes done regularly during your lunch hour will yield results! Exercise is one of the best investments you can make with your time to ensure an independent, active older adult lifestyle.

Uche's Story

I know all about the word "busy"! Not only do I maintain a busy dental practice, Kary and I spend several hours per week researching and preparing speeches, articles, and ideas for books. We travel frequently (the kids come too) for speaking engagements and, of course, we are devoted parents. Since the children were born, we have not been able to be at the gym every day of the week, but we have learned ways to incorporate the whole family in active lifestyle practices like family walks, playing at the local park, and enjoying home-cooked, organic meals.

Kary and I take turns going to the gym. I participate in a weekly yoga class, and every morning I perform about 10 minutes of yoga stretches that I learned from class, which gets me ready for the day. I train with weights and cardiovascular equipment three times per week. These sessions include a moderate-intensity 15-minute warm-up on cardio equipment, circuit weight training that keeps my heart rate elevated, and a 10-minute relaxation activity at the end.

Health Miracle

If both parents make fitness a must, then you increase the likelihood of your child being physically active to 70 percent!

Do You Have the Time?

Those who think they have no time for bodily exercise will sooner or later have to find time for illness.
　—Edward Stanley

Here's a little secret: You don't find time, you make time! Remember, time is a non-renewable resource, so value it instead of wasting it. Your valuable time should be accounted for—you are the president of "You, Inc." Time is the great equalizer! Rich man, poor man, beggar man, and thief: we all have our allotted 24 hours per day, seven days per week. What separates the doers from the watchers is the effective use of that time.

There are 168 hours in a week, and everyone on the planet has the same amount of time. What makes the difference is how each of us uses that time. Our quality of life is a direct result of what we do with the hours we have been given. Can you spare half an hour to 45 minutes three times a week for exercise? Not too much to ask, considering that's barely 1 percent of our time in a week!

Some say the best time to start a fitness regimen is when you are young. We say the next best time is *now!* Get the message? If you are thinking about something, then it is time to *take action!* T-N-T. (That means Today, Not Tomorrow!) The results could literally blow you away!

Health Miracle

Building your back muscles with resistance training helps you in many other areas aside from looking good at the beach. Working on those hard-to-see muscles will make you stronger in every task—gardening, housekeeping, playing with the kids, etc. Another bonus is better posture, which helps you carry yourself better and protects your spine from injury.

Time As an Investment

There are only two things you can do with time—spend it or invest it. If you spend it, it's gone forever. When invested, it creates a lifetime residual.
    —James Arthur Ray

Many North Americans are working more and enjoying less free time. The following is a list of some easy ways for you to free up more time for your health, and get into the best investment you will ever make.

1. Check and respond to your e-mails once or twice per day.

2. Shorten your paper trail. We each get almost 3,000 pieces of mail a year. Our recommendation? Touch each piece of mail only once, and ask yourself if it ought to be thrown out or dealt with.

3. Work harder at work. It is amazing that only 60 percent of our 8-hour days are productive. Try increasing your pace instead of staying longer at the office or taking work home.

4. Simplify your life. Downsize the number of things you have to look after. De-junk your home. Having less stuff means more time to enjoy what's really important—health and fitness and the special people in your life.

5. Start a family calendar. We keep a corkboard with 12 calendar pages posted in our home office, so we can view our major events, trips, and goals for the year. And, we schedule in our fitness! A year can fly by quickly. Why not make each day count? These calendar pages can be saved forever as documentation of your family's accomplishments!

Health Miracle

Exercise reduces one of the major risk factors for strokes and heart attacks: arterial inflammation.

Health Miracle Activities

1. Think of at least one way that you could manage time better, thus freeing up more of it for health and fitness.

_____

2. Write down three reasons or excuses that prevent you from acting on your health goals. It will put them into perspective maybe for the first time. You may even start to think of how those reasons or excuses have affected your life. Remember, it has been said that awareness alone can start the process of change. By identifying your excuses, you will be taking the first step toward better outcomes!

(a) _____

(b) _____

(c) _____

3. How will you and your loved ones benefit if you stop making these excuses?

_____

Chapter 9

To be seventy years young is sometimes far more cheerful and hopeful than to be forty years old.
—Oliver Wendell Holmes

Active Older Adult

The man who views the world at 50 the same way as he did at 20 has wasted 30 years of his life.
—Mohammed Ali

Richard Bach said, "Here is the test to find whether your mission on Earth is finished: if you're alive, it isn't." Maybe this is why we refer to the latter part of life as the golden years: instead of conforming to preconceived notions of old age, you have the option of reinventing yourself at any age!

According to Dr. William Bortz of Stanford University Medical School, there are only two scientifically proven ways for humans to lower the risks of age-related diseases and to look and feel younger: having a healthy diet and engaging in regular exercise. This is a powerful promise for anyone who started this book with feelings of fear about the aging process.

A seminar attendee once approached us during a break and shared his personal testimony about living an active life: "I enjoy getting up early and walking over to the YMCA with my wife. Both of us are early risers, but instead of sitting around the house wishing we could sleep longer, we made a decision several years ago to get over to the Y and swim some laps first thing in the morning. We are both in our seventies and I have arthritis, but the brisk walk gets me warmed up. And the 45 minutes in the pool make me forget about my condition and I feel great for the rest of the day!"

> *If you don't renovate,*
> *things deteriorate!*

Can you picture that couple power walking down the road to their YMCA for their morning swim? You really are as young as you think you are.

Health Miracle

The human body has 600 muscles and 200 bones. It yearns for activity and movement. And it was built to last! Steven Austad, of the University of Idaho, says that the first person to reach 150 years of age may be alive as you are reading this book.

Fixed Beliefs

Anyone who stops learning is old, whether at 20 or 80. Anyone who keeps learning stays young. The greatest thing in life is to keep your mind young.
—Henry Ford

The power of fixed beliefs was illustrated profoundly in a university experiment where two species of fish (predator and prey) were separated in a tank by a glass wall for several weeks. The predators kept butting themselves against the wall at first, trying to get to their prey. Eventually they stopped trying, realizing that they could not cross the boundary of the glass wall. When the wall finally was removed, the fish lived out the rest of their lives without crossing the imaginary border. Like the fish with the perceived barrier, many people maintain old limiting beliefs that have outworn their use. Some people live out their lives without ever challenging them and never venture into new territory.

You may have heard of Roger Bannister, the first person to run a mile in under 4 minutes. Prior to 1954, this was believed to be an impossible human feat, but Roger ignored the fixed beliefs of exercise physiologists and scientists of the day. Interestingly enough, within the first few years after Roger broke through that limit, many others repeated his performance. This story is only one of many that prove fixed beliefs can limit our physical potential.

> ### *Health Miracle*
>
> **Researchers studied two groups of recent retirees for four years. An exercising group maintained nearly the same level of blood flow in the brain, while the inactive group had a significant decrease.**

Getting Beyond the Fixed Beliefs

I have only one wrinkle and I'm sitting on it!
   —Jeanne Calment (who lived to 122 years of age)

Many people have such rigid fixed beliefs about getting older. They see it as a time of disease and deterioration. Negative self-talk reinforces the following thoughts:

"Look at all these wrinkles."
"I just don't have the memory I used to."
"I wish I was young again."
"My bones hurt."
"I'm no good to anyone."

These fixed ideas can limit our expectations for our senior years. Yes, it used to be a time of ailments, nursing homes, and pining away for the good old days. But now, with the knowledge and use of fitness, nutrition, and mind-body medicine, the experience of growing older has radically changed.

> **Did You Know?**
> *In 2008 there are 500 million people over age 65.*
> *By 2050 that total will increase threefold.*

Can we halt the aging process? Or, even better, reverse it? First, we have to get away from old, fixed, stale ideas about aging, and we need to believe that life is still worth living. Research has shown that losing the will to live is more fatal than cancer or cardiovascular disease. A new outlook on disease and prevention is needed. British historian George Trevelyan, once said, "I have two doctors, my left leg and my right."

Life is no longer just about survival; our society values contribution, personal fulfillment, and achievement. People have the luxury of more leisure time to think and ponder when they reach their fifties and sixties. For some, pondering may lead to panicking, and panicking creates the fear that immobilizes you. Being immobilized means you are more likely to stay put. And if that happens, you eventually wake up one day and do a little review of all your choices and wonder why you haven't accomplished more.

Health Miracle

You can shave 10–20 years off your physiological age just by improving your aerobic capacity 15–20 percent! Try brisk walking or cycling to boost oxygen consumption.

The Age of Reinvention

Far better to dare mighty things, to win glorious triumphs even though checkered by failures, than to rank with those poor spirits who neither enjoy nor suffer much because they live in the gray twilight that knows neither victory nor defeat.
—Theodore Roosevelt

The ideas of renewal and personal development after age 55 were not so important 100 years ago because people, on average, did not live much past 55. Now we are living well into our eighties and beyond. And the research shows that quality of life and independent living are possible if you engage in a healthy lifestyle. Today's healthy seniors are the pioneers of the new aging: they are going to university, working in and out of their homes, studying new languages, engaging in physical activity, using the Internet, and discovering new hobbies.

For some people, growing older doesn't mean living with lower expectations. They look to the future with anticipation versus fear.

> *How old would you be if you did not know how old you were?*

If you look, you can find people in your life who exemplify the possibility that growing older doesn't necessarily mean failing health and reduced vitality. These people are reinventing themselves by trying new things and keeping their outlook fresh. If you can't think of any, read some biographies or watch Biography on the Arts and Entertainment Channel.

Aging can bring many benefits like insight, wisdom, spirituality, and more time for the pursuit of your passions. Would you like a different way to look at birthdays? Instead of sadly checking off another year, and dreading the next, try the following advice. Reflect back on the experiences you have enjoyed and endured on the planet to date. Make a commitment to utilize all of your wisdom in the coming year and create the best year of your life!

Inspiring People

I think like a young person and, although I try to keep myself fit and active, I won't be taking desperate measures like face-lifts and plastic surgery. I'm a great believer in letting nature take its course and living with what I've been given.
    —Sharon Stone

- In 2008 John McCain won the Republican nomination for president of the U.S. at age 71.

- Claude Monet was 73 when he began work on his famous water lily paintings.

- John Glenn came out of retirement to re-enter the world of space travel at age 78.

- Nobel prizewinner Albert Schweitzer took up medicine in midlife. He worked into his eighties in his famous African hospital.

- Famous artist Grandma Moses took up painting in her late seventies.

- At age 73, Thomas Edison started the campaign for the Naval Research laboratory.

- Oscar winner Shirley MacLaine, in her sixties, trekked 500 miles in 30 days on a spiritual pilgrimage in Spain.

- Ronald Reagan became president of the United States in his late sixties. He went on to become one of the most charismatic world leaders of the twentieth century.

- Harland Sanders, the founder of Kentucky Fried Chicken, started his multimillion-dollar business at 62!

- Harrison Ford, in his sixties, did many of his own stunts in the 2008 release of the Indiana Jones movie series.

- Justice Oliver Wendell Holmes was writing Supreme Court decisions at 90. When president-elect Franklin Roosevelt paid a visit to Holmes in 1933, Holmes was reading Plato in Greek. When Roosevelt asked why, the 92-year-old Holmes answered, "Why, to improve my mind."

- Arnold Schwarzenegger reinvented himself for the third time as a politician and began his second term as Governor of California in his sixties!

For more inspiration and information, visit:
www.growingbolder.com
www.lifelongfitnessalliance.org
www.thirdage.com

Health Miracle

You can decrease the risk of Alzheimer's by about 50 percent with regular exercise. Exercise helps to break down the sticky proteins in the brain that are linked to this disease.

Adding Life to Your Years

One must never lose time in vainly regretting the past nor in complaining about the changes which cause us discomfort, for change is the very essence of life.
　　—Anatole France, French poet, journalist, and novelist

Scientists who study aging have a term called "biomarkers." These are not body paints! These are changes like sagging skin, failing vision, deteriorating hearing, slackening muscles, weakening immunity, and dying brain cells (starting at age 30 if there's no intervention).

　　On the other hand, Walter Bortz, M.D., author of *We Live Too Short and Die Too Long*, says the human body has real renewable qualities: by taking responsibility for ourselves, taking charge of important areas in our lives, exercising regularly, and eating with sound nutrition, we can extend our life expectancy.

　　Ben Douglas, Ph.D., author of *Ageless: Living Younger Longer*, reports that our bodies are meant to live approximately five times the age of our sexual maturity. In other words, human bodies are designed to last well over a century. You are *meant* to live many more years than you have been led to believe, and many of the determining factors are in your control.

Health Miracle

A Tufts University study showed an increase of 1 percent of bone density in the hips and spine of strength-training women and a decrease of 2.5 percent for a sedentary group over the course of one year.

Live Long, Live Well!

Youth is not a period of one's life. It's a state of mind, an effort of will, a quality of the imagination, an emotional intensity. . . . [W]e only grow old when we abandon our ideals.
　　—Douglas MacArthur

There are many healthy habits that can add years to your life: a positive attitude, physical activity, cessation of smoking, supplementation, stress-reduction activities, and better food choices can all affect the aging process. We have compiled the following lifestyle tips to give you a head start.

- **Change your self-talk.** Refrain from using statements like: "My old bones." "You can't teach an old dog new tricks!" "I'm too old!" "It's all downhill from here." "I only have a few good years left." In *The Secret*, Dr. Ben Johnson explains: "We are now entering the era of energy medicine. Everything in the Universe has a frequency and all you have to do is change a frequency or create an opposite frequency. That's how easy it is to change anything in the world."

- **Make yourself indispensable.** By volunteering your time and energy, you can add value to any cause. It is one of the simplest ways to make a difference. It doesn't cost anything, and there are an endless number of organizations and causes that are in need of people like you. Volunteering with youth can be extremely rewarding and mutually beneficial.

- **Start something new.** Having projects that you are actively working on adds passion to your daily existence. Howard E. Hill, in *Energizing the 12 Powers of the Mind*, reported that having ongoing projects at any age is a definite way to escape mediocrity. We believe the rewards and benefits will ripple out to all areas of your life. There is an old saying that goes "There is not much to do but bury a man when the last of his dreams are dead."

- **Change your surroundings.** Colors, textures, brightness, open spaces can all help shape the way you feel. Why not take charge of your environment, so it refreshes and rejuvenates you? Paint your rooms in bright, cheerful colors. Buy some beautiful plants. Did you know that houseplants can improve the air quality in your home? Philodendrons and spider plants are the most effective air cleaners, according to a NASA study.

- **Stay sexually active!** Studies have shown that couples who maintain an active sex life have more emotional, mental, and physical enjoyment as they age. At a basic level, regular exercise improves physical fitness and self-esteem, and sexual functioning is related to those areas.

- **Do good deeds!** Operating from the goodness of your heart adds life to your years and years to your life. The best-seller *Random Acts of Kindness* tells of the karmic energy that comes as a by-product of doing good deeds for others.

- **Keep your mind flexible and open.** Make an effort to surround yourself with others who are open and positive. Attitudes are extremely contagious. If you regularly get together with people who discuss tragedies in the newspaper, recent illness, and their worries, your psyche will suffer. Avoid hardening of the mental arteries!

- **Take advantage of the Law of Forgiveness.** In order to enjoy excellent health and peace of mind, one must be able to forgive and forget. Holding grudges may hold anyone back from ever achieving his or her true potential and ultimate joy in life. Spiritual gurus Marianne Williamson and Louise Hay say that forgiveness is the first step to healing any area of your life.

- **Smile more.** If you frown or scowl a lot, you will create vertical wrinkles between your eyebrows. Repetitive expressions, which tell of sadness, suffering, and anger, can distort the skin, leaving permanent reminders. Always remember that a smile is energizing. We liken it to instant Botox—without the side-effects!

- **Wear a baseball cap and/or sunscreen.** The sun's ultraviolet rays affect the collagen layers in our skin, causing us to look older faster.

- **Don't follow yo-yo diets.** Weight fluctuations stretch the skin, and the skin has a difficult time regaining its appearance each time the weight is lost and regained.

- **Wear properly fitting, comfortable shoes.** If you buy poor-fitting shoes or wear old, outworn ones, you will harm your feet and cause deformities.

- **Ask your optometrist about eye exercises.** The eye lens stiffens with age. Dr. Deepak Chopra, in his audio program "Magical Mind, Magical Body," shares with his readers a series of eye exercises that may be used to lessen the effect of aging on the eye muscles.

- **Take care of your teeth and gums.** Did you know that the bacteria in the mouth have been implicated in certain cardiac conditions? Research has shown that daily flossing and regular dental visits can possibly increase our lifespan by six years.

- **Walk every day.** Aim for 30 minutes in total, either all at once or in increments throughout the day. Walking helps to increase the synovial fluid in the joints, which is the lubricant that protects you from joint conditions like arthritis. Walking is a true miracle exercise that is affordable and easy.

Health Miracle

In the third decade of life, the human brain gradually begins to lose tissue. Cognitive performance declines with this loss. Studies have shown that losses in brain tissue were substantially reduced as a function of cardiovascular fitness. The benefits of exercise on the brain health of older adults is an exciting area of research!

Exercise Enhances Life

Do not fear death so much, but rather the inadequate life.
    —Bertolt Brecht

The role of exercise is vital to aging gracefully. Basically, if you don't use it, you lose it! People who tend to have a couch potato lifestyle when they are younger often end up as mashed potatoes when they are older. Did you know that you are losing muscle mass as you age? Every year you lose about 1 percent of your muscle mass if you don't perform some type of resistance activity. Less muscle mass means less fat-burning potential, which leads to increased fat storage. Of course, this can lead to a myriad of problems and eventually to loss of independence.

Muscle is a very active, highly functioning tissue. When you have more muscle and less fat on your body, you have increased ability to enjoy all of life's activities. Lifting weights or resistance training for as little as 20 minutes, two times per week will protect you from diseases of inactivity, like osteoporosis. In addition, aerobic exercise like walking, cycling, swimming, and dancing will protect and strengthen your heart and lungs. Top this off with a stretching and flexibility program and you will stay limber, resist injury, and feel youthful. Try looking under "Health" or "Fitness" in the Yellow Pages to find information about trainers, gyms, and community clubs. Reduced muscle tissue and inflexibility are two of the major reasons the elderly are at risk for debilitating broken hips and other fractures due to falls.

The benefits of exercise are numerous, and it is never too late to get started. In one study, 300 hospital patients (over 70 years of age) were divided into two groups after an extended stay. Only one of the groups was given an exercise program to follow. It was found that people in this group were able to go about their daily activities much better than those who didn't follow the exercise program.

A personal trainer told us about one of his clients who had truly amazed his medical doctors and family. The man was turning 80 and required a walker due to a lifetime of inactivity, which led to muscle wasting, weakness, and decreased confidence. His doctor told him that if he did not start building some strength, he would need a wheelchair soon. The man took action and met with the trainer. He started a re-sistance-training program, combined with aerobic training, and made improvements quickly. One year later the man had not only sold his walker, he was out jogging in the street!

A recent study from McMaster University in Hamilton, Ontario, put healthy seniors on a one-hour, twice-weekly resistance-training program for six months. The average age of the seniors was 70 and they had never participated in weight training before. The seniors experienced a 50 percent improvement in strength and reported great benefits in their personal lives. Even more exciting, this study also examined the cellular mitochondria, which are typically depleted in older people. Associate Professor Dr. Mark Tarnopolsky reported a change in the condition of the mitochondria: after the six-month program, the mitochondria of the seniors resembled those found in women and men between 25–35 years of age! This is extremely significant since the mitochondria fuel activity in cells. Perhaps resistance training is the "fountain of youth"!

> *A gene that produces a protein that stimulates osteoblasts to build bone is turned on by weight lifting!*

Regular exercise has positive effects on a number of medical conditions that have been associated with the elderly:

1. Lowers diabetes risk
2. Helps manage stress
3. Helps prevent osteoporosis
4. Increases good cholesterol and decreases blood pressure
5. Decreases joint stiffness and increases mobility
6. Decreases the risk of many cancers
7. Helps regulate hormone levels during menopause
8. Increases memory and other mental abilities
9. Decreases osteoarthritis and joint pain
10. Helps control body weight

Uche's Story

As a practising dentist, I am continually inspired by the stories I hear. I always ask my older, healthy patients what they are doing to keep themselves young. One 66-year-old gentleman told me that he was inspired to take action while visiting a friend in a cancer-treatment facility. He was overwhelmed by the number of people in the unit. He noticed how frail and vulnerable they looked, some hooked up to oxygen tanks and others looking as if they had no reason to live. He left the hospital and vowed to start taking better care *of himself and to help others in the process. He convinced several friends that they needed to do something, so they started training and fundraising for the annual Ride for the Cure in Toronto. His group has raised over $83,000 to date! I assumed that he had always been a cyclist, but once again he surprised me when he told me that he hadn't ridden a bike since his teens. He had to go out and buy one!*

Health Miracle

Researchers from Tufts University in Boston had frail 90-year-olds participate in eight weeks of resistance training. These older adults had mid-thigh muscle size increases of around 9 percent and averaged muscle-strength gains of 174 percent!

Balance Training

It is better to wear out than to rust out.
  —Richard Cumberland

By training your body to work in circumstances that are unstable, you can condition it to prevent many falls. For people over 65, falling is the number-one cause of accidental death. An excellent idea would be to hire a gymnastics instructor or a martial arts instructor to teach you how to fall correctly.

Balance Tips:

- Use dumbbells instead of machines for most of your strength training. This forces you to learn how to lift and balance the weights. Many popular strength-training exercises involve balance: e.g., lunges, step-ups, and squats.

- Practise standing in a safe area with your eyes closed. Gradually increase the amount of time you are able to keep your eyes closed.

If you progress rapidly, try doing the same exercise on one foot. Stand close to a stable object like a wall, couch, or heavy chair in case you need to steady yourself.

- Try doing some of your standing exercises on one leg to improve your body awareness, or proprioception. Use lighter resistance or no resistance when trying these exercises.

- Using unstable equipment like stability balls, balance boards, and Bosu balls is an advanced way to build your balance.

- Try yoga and tai chi. They are marvelous forms of exercise that have the unique ability to help you age well. The deliberate movements and poses have thousands of years of proven history behind them. They will help with balance, breathing, flexibility and strength.

Health Miracle

Improving muscular strength and flexibility can also prevent back pain and reduce the risk of falls.

Nutrition

One who eats whole food will be strong and healthy.
— Okinawan proverb

Remember to consult your physician before making any changes to your nutrition or supplementation program.

Following sound nutritional principles is one of the easiest ways to *age-proof* yourself. Our basic nutrition advice in chapters 4 and 5 applies to all ages. Put to use, it will help with your quest for a long and healthy life. We have also compiled a list of nutritional recommendations specifically for active older adults.

- Drink water to keep your kidneys in shape. Kidneys lose function naturally at the rate of about 1 percent per year. Drinking at least six to eight glasses per day becomes even more important as we get older.

- Include green tea several times per day. It has been shown to have potent antioxidant properties and has less caffeine than black tea.

- Stay current with what's new in nutrition. There is always new literature on healthy eating and its effects on our bodies. Be a lifelong learner, and stay on top of recent discoveries in the world of nutrition.

- Include more of the Top Foods from Chapter 5. These foods are the cancer-fighting, health-supporting nutrition powerhouses!

- Include a green drink in your daily ritual. We love greens+ bone builder from Genuine Health to maintain an alkaline, bone-supportive environment in your body.

- Invest in a good probiotic supplement to increase the good bacteria in your gut and reduce inflammation. This is especially important during and after a treatment with antibiotics, which kill good and bad bacteria.

- Invest in a good-quality omega-3 fish oil supplement. Our choice is o3mega from Genuine Health.

- Eat less animal fats, fried foods, and fats that are solid at room temperature. These fats contain more LDL cholesterol. Heart experts have defined LDL cholesterol as "less desirable" because it gums up the lining of blood vessels. HDL cholesterol is desirable because it is transported to the liver where it is either sent out as waste or used in important hormone production. HDL may actually help pick up LDL cholesterol in arteries and clear it from the body. Immediately following a workout, HDL can be temporarily increased by up to 20 percent.

- Invest in one or two sessions with a naturopathic doctor or registered holistic nutritionist. It may cost $80 to $150 per visit, although many health care plans provide coverage. The individualized information can save you from years of uncertainty about nutritional deficiencies, food allergies, or intolerances.

- Have you ever eaten to the point of having to unbutton your pants? UCLA's Dr. Roy Walford reports that he could extend the lifespan of mice five times by feeding them less food. His research points to the concept that overeating puts a strain on the human body and shortens life. He recommends that you eat to a level of comfort, and put your fork away! Dr. Deepak Chopra also agrees with this concept. His findings suggest eating until the stomach is full taxes your system unnecessarily. Because the stomach is a muscular bag, it is best filled up only to two-thirds and the rest left empty for digestive action. Less energy used for digestion means more energy for other functions in the body, such as mental tasks, physical movement, and repair of injuries.

Health Miracle

Increasing your fitness level has been shown to reduce some menopausal symptoms, such as night sweats and hot flashes.

Health Miracle Activity

Resource
International Council of Active Aging: www.icaa.cc

Close your eyes and picture in your mind an 80-year-old couple. What do they look like, and what kinds of things are they doing? What is their posture like, and how healthy are they? Do this now before you read the next sentence.

What you have just imagined is indicative of your beliefs about old age. Ultimately, with your present beliefs, this is how you will look and feel at 80. If you did not like your vision, then you must take responsibility now. Beginning to let go of those preconceived notions of what one should look and feel like at a certain age is the first step toward growing older with joy and anticipation instead of fear and trepidation.

Chapter 10

There are two types of people—anchors and motors. You want to lose the anchors and get with the motors because the motors are going somewhere and they're having more fun. The anchors will just drag you down.

—Wyland, world-renowned marine artist

Who Are You Flocking With?

Men take on the nature, the habits, and the power of thought of those with whom they associate.
—Napoleon Hill

Have you ever heard the old saying "Birds of a feather flock together?" The leading experts in human performance tell us that if we want to enjoy more success, we'd better start spending time with successful people. Why? Because our relationships have tremendous influence on our thoughts and behaviors. Relationships are the foundation of everything you set out to achieve. We intuitively know this information to be true. Just look at any parent's protectiveness when it comes to his or her children's friends!

It has been said that life satisfaction is mainly dependent on the relationships you have formed over the years with family, friends, and people in your community (church, work, etc.). Studies have shown that reaching out to your support group can reduce stress. If you are helping someone else—or being helped—you can raise positive hormones like oxytocin, the bonding hormone. Dr. Christiane Northrup explains, in *Mother-Daughter Wisdom*, that high levels of oxytocin help us to seek out more friendships and it also promotes relaxation.

If we spend the majority of our time with people who enjoy active lifestyles, it's easier to start incorporating healthy practices into our own lives. Did you know that psychological research has shown that we can only admire traits in others that we ourselves possess? In other words, if you admire a friend's disciplined pursuit of fitness, then you yourself have the potential to develop that same discipline. If you didn't have this potential, you wouldn't even notice it in others.

So, if you want more health in your life, start hanging around with healthy people! You can join a gym, recreation center, or club. Sign up for a class and arrive early and linger afterwards. Attend a weekend yoga retreat, a fitness clinic, or a health seminar.

Most people who are successful in an area of their life like to share information and mentor others. Be open and willing to taking advantage of this. You may be surprised to hear someone's story is similar to your own. There are many people who have overcome tragic circumstances and gone on to have great prosperity and happiness. For the cost of a coffee or lunch you can lose yourself in someone else's story and learn new insights to assist you in your journey.

Health Miracle

Research by Professor Shelley E. Taylor, Ph.D., shows that we have a built-in health enhancer when we engage in "tend and befriend" habits. These nurturing behaviors enhance immunity and protect against heart disease.

Energy Drainers

Keep away from people who belittle your ambitions. Small people always do that, but the really great make you feel that you, too, can become great.
—Mark Twain

Do you have friends or family members who rarely have anything positive to say? Have you noticed that they zap your energy and leave you feeling drained and uncomfortable? They are the people in your life who seem to have a knack for letting everyone around them know what *isn't* possible. Remember these people who tell you what's impossible are often the people who cannot imagine new, healthy lifestyle habits in their own lives. They are simply projecting their own fears, inabilities, or feelings of inadequacy onto you.

Inspirational speaker and corporate trainer Les Brown has a great response to these folks: "What you think about me is none of my business!"

It would be fantastic to be able to replay these words in our minds whenever we are on the receiving end of another's negative broadcast. Everyone is entitled to his or her opinion, but the key word here is *opinion*. It only becomes a fact if we buy into it.

Of course, everyone deserves a second chance, but when do you draw the line? Energy Drainers constantly complain about their lives, but never take any action. In addition, they may constantly remind you of your failures, possibly thwarting your attempts to move ahead. They may even try to convince you that you should be satisfied with the way things are.

Health Miracle

Regular exercise is an admirable lifestyle habit, so if you are looking for your soul mate or new people to flock with, try your local gym or put on some cologne and go for a run! By taking care of yourself, you're indirectly saying, "I'm valuable." And the person with a good self-concept is possibly someone who's worth getting to know!

Energy Givers

You are the average of the five people you spend the most time with.
—Jim Rohn

Energy Givers are those people in our lives who challenge us to meet our full potential. They focus on our strengths (which we sometimes do not see) and give unconditional support and love, even when we're engulfed by the darkness of self-doubt.

There are many benefits to spending time with the Energy Givers in our lives. Their enthusiasm for their own projects and interests is contagious. They are passionately involved in activities and careers they love. Here are eight more characteristics of Energy Givers:

1. They have an unconscious competence about their actions—they make things look easy.

2. They live their lives without seeking approval and they are easy to be with.

3. Their faces glow with an unmistakable light: they stand out in a crowd, and their smiles are contagious.

4. They look for the positive qualities in others, and they find it easy to give compliments.

5. They make you feel important by giving you their full attention when you are with them.

6. They are committed to their own self-improvement and the improvement of society.

7. They usually have interesting stories and insights into the human condition.

8. They are open-minded.

How does a person become an Energy Giver in the world of fitness? There are many ways. You can begin by taking care of yourself. By following sound nutritional practices, getting sufficient rest, and staying active, you are in a better position to positively influence others in your sphere. Become known for encouraging and supporting others' efforts to get fit.

A new commitment to health and fitness is fragile in its beginning stages. It is very easy to get off track. Did you know that it takes 21–30 days for a new behavior to become a habit? In the early stages, it is very important to strengthen your own resolve and nurture your new healthy choices daily. This may mean sharing only with Energy Givers, not everyone around you!

If you do not have any Energy Givers or positive role models in your life, then read about them! An uplifting biography can be a great way to tune into the mindset of people who have reached the summit. Let your imagination work wonders while you read! With every autobiography and biography, we are given an intimate look into the life of a person we may never get a chance to meet. Miracles await all those who can make reading an integral part of their lives.

Health Miracle

A health study in the community of Tecumseh, Michigan, found that men who participate in group activities and have more friends and better relationships with relatives show lower levels of stroke, cancer, heart disease, and lung disease.

A Healing Network

One cannot live in this world without the support of others.
—Okinawan proverb

In our stressful, technological world, social connections are especially important. Going through a major life event alone can be one of the most stressful times in your life. It is key to make healthy, supportive connections with other people. Ask yourself the question, "Where are my current friends leading me?" It is important to have relationships with people who inspire, uplift, or bring out the best in you. Don't think for a moment that you can spend time with people and not be affected or influenced by their beliefs.

A surefire way to gain the support of your friends and family is to constantly focus on the positive aspects of your newfound health regime. We understand that this might not be easy in the early days when you first experience the soreness of unused muscles and you are getting used to the new routine of stopping at the gym instead of the coffee shop on your way to work! But believe us—your circle of friends will pay close attention to the energy you are giving off and they will reciprocate with more of the same. So, if you constantly complain and moan, your loved ones will wonder why you are bothering with this new lifestyle and they will advise you to quit. On the other hand, if you share the pride you feel and the self-confidence you are gaining, your family and friends will most likely support your endeavors. Who knows? They might even ask to join you!

Enlist support from friends, family, a personal trainer, a nutritionist, and your other health care providers. Take responsibility for your relationships and treat them like gold! Be willing to support and help others, and expect the same in return.

Health Miracle

The *Journal of the American Medical Association* reported a study that exposed over 250 healthy volunteers to a cold virus. Amazingly, those who had greater social networks and more close relationships were more resistant to the virus! Only 35 percent of this group caught the cold, versus 62 percent of the group with poor social networks.

The Power of Two

To be able to find joy in another's joy: that is the secret of happiness.
—George Bernanos

You are about 35 percent more likely to stick to a fitness regime with a training partner.

Once you harness the "power of two," there is no stopping what you can do! Stephen Covey's concept of synergy states that when two people come together in harmony, a more effective outcome will be achieved than either could have accomplished alone. 1+1 can add up to 2, but if you look at it with synergy in mind, 1+1 can become 11. Here are some tips for you to share with your significant other or workout buddy:

- Discuss your mental picture of health and fitness. Do not judge or argue about whose version is more accurate. An important defining trait of any close and fulfilling relationship is finding and building common ground.

- Assist each other in rediscovering an unrealized wish from childhood. You can then nurture and support a long-forgotten dream to dance or to run a marathon. Hey, ladies, if you are looking to improve your fitness level and your husband or boyfriend is not interested, maybe the best thing to do is to find out what sport he liked when he was in high school. If it was hockey, then buy some skates and take him to the nearest rink! Hey, guys, if your wife or girlfriend is not too interested in weight training and you would like to try something active together, then maybe it's time for the ballroom-dancing lessons she's been hinting about for the past two years!

- If you have a reluctant significant other or friend, your desire to help may simply be put into action by setting a good example. Never give up on them! As you begin to notice your own positive benefits, share them with your spouse or friend. If you see a glimmer of interest, then encourage it and ask them to join you.

- Give each other praise anytime you take a healthy step forward. By making deposits in your emotional bank accounts, you encourage each other to take further action. Long before toned muscles appear and excess pounds disappear, you can genuinely nurture and appreciate each other's efforts. This is behavior modification at its best!

- Be flexible in scheduling your shared fitness activities. Flexibility in your scheduling is as important as working on the flexibility of your body.

Ted and Terri's Story

After you spoke to our study club in Kansas, I thought I would wait a few months to see if the lessons you taught were still having an effect on my life. After about three months, your presentation had a dramatic effect on both me and my wife. Before we heard you speak, we were both overweight, had a very poor diet, and the only exercise we got was walking to the refrigerator. My wife was on two medications for high blood pressure and we both battled high cholesterol. The only plan we had in our lives was planning what we were going to have for dinner. That has changed, thanks to you guys.

We knew we had to make changes in our lives, but really didn't know how to go about it and we really needed someone to ignite our motivation. You were the spark that we needed. Thankfully, my wife and I both heard you because change is much easier with a partner. We are now aware of what we eat. No more bread in restaurants, smaller portions, no empty-calorie foods. Instead of coming home from work and eating a bag of chips and a handful of cookies, we come home and eat a handful of nuts and make a salad. If it's too cold to walk outside, we walk on our treadmill. My wife has done a better job of writing down her goals, but one of my goals is to finish my goal list, and I will.

(continued)

My wife now only takes a low-dose diuretic for her blood pressure, her triglycerides are a third of what they were, and her cholesterol is back to normal. I have lost 15 pounds and my wife has lost 10. None of our clothes fit anymore. I feel like I have more energy and I'm more productive at work. I have talked to others that attended the seminar and they are seeing similar results. You have really made a major change in our lives. The lessons you taught are now a lifestyle for us, not just something we tried for a couple of weeks and gave up on.

Your Family

The best way to inspire your children to develop into the kind of adults you dream of them becoming is to become the kind of adult you want them to be.
—Robin Sharma

Your environment plays a part in how you think and act. Create a warm, loving, calm environment for your children. It is very important for children to see their parents taking care of themselves and enjoying life. Shakti Gawain, in her book *Living in the Light*, says that for many parents, having children is an easy excuse to neglect their own needs. Fitness is usually one of the first things to go when schedules are hectic.

But consider this: Children are masters of observation. If they see their parents enjoying fitness activities, they are more likely to make it part of their everyday lives. Practising sound nutrition and engaging in fun fitness activities with your children could add an entirely new dimension to your own enjoyment. Remember that you are a leader when you become a parent! Try the following suggestions to rejuvenate your family's health profile:

- Make family mealtime a time for sharing goals and achievements. Discuss plans for family outings and activities. The family that plays together, stays together!

- Create a few fitness rituals. We love to walk to a small pond after dinner, where our youngest really enjoys seeing the baby ducks and geese and other pond wildlife. Every Sunday, Daddy takes the kids swimming while Mommy works out in the gym. The kids love looking up and waving to Mom through the window of the viewing area!

- If you have small children, shop with them and explain the names of the fruits and vegetables. It is amazing how much they remember if you make it fun.

- Pack healthy snacks for your children every time you leave the house. Don't buy into the temptation to give them "junk food" just because you are out. Young children will eat what is presented if they are truly

> *Your children are 70 percent more likely to become active adults if both parents are physically active.*

hungry. Bring several options. We use hard-boiled eggs, cut-up vegetables, raisins, grapes, berries, "pancakes" (made from eggs, oatmeal, and cinnamon), rice cakes, and organic cheeses.

Health Miracle Activities

1. Make a list of all the people with whom you regularly spend time (at least once per week).

   _____

   _____

   _____

   _____

2. Put an "EG" for Energy Giver beside all the people who enhance your life by being positive and nurturing. In other words, when you leave a conversation or meeting with these people, you feel good. Put an "ED" for Energy Drainer beside all the people who are negative forces in your life. In other words, when you leave a conversation or meeting with these people, you feel drained or upset.

3. Look over your list and make a commitment to spend more quality time with your EGs and less time or no time with your EDs.

4. Now this one might be a little more difficult. Think of the people on whom you have a direct influence. Would they consider you an Energy Drainer or Energy Giver? How can you increase your Energy Giver status?

Chapter 11

Life is like riding a bicycle. To keep your balance you must keep moving.
> —Albert Einstein

Desperately Seeking Balance

We've got a thousand different diagnoses and diseases out there. They're just the weak link. They're all the result of one thing: stress. If you put enough stress on the chain and you put enough stress on the system, then one of the links break.
—Dr. Ben Johnson

Everyone seems to be searching for balance these days. Your career is demanding of your time. Your children want you. You have five favorite shows to watch. E-mails beckon you to the laptop. Newspapers demand reading. Then there is that party to plan.

Calgon, take me away!

Do you remember that line from the commercial? But who has time these days to draw a bath and take a dip when the UPS driver is ringing your doorbell and your cell phone is buzzing in your gym bag?

Balance is a nice concept, yet how realistic is it to think that we might actually achieve a completely harmonious state of being with no stress; no pressures from work, home, or friends; and with no unforeseen road bumps or blocks impeding our progress? Sounds like a bit of a pipe dream! And maybe even a little bit boring! James Ray, best-selling author of *Harmonic Wealth*, reported that balance is bogus and that people need to look at it differently. Everything is not going to be in balance. Rather, at any given time, you are focused on one area and that takes the lead. Then at another time in your life, spirituality may get more of your attention and the other areas are out of the limelight.

We love this concept because we feel that whenever you work on anything of significance in your life, it has a ripple effect on all other areas. John F. Kennedy said, "When the tide comes in, all ships rise together."

In this chapter we deal only with balance as it relates to your physical health and well-being, the basis for all other forms of excellence. So we will start with the main deterrent to feeling balanced: stress and the consequences of stress.

Not All Stress Is Bad Stress

The human journey involves not just a spiritual awakening but the development of all levels of our being—spiritual, mental, emotional, and physical—and the integration of all these aspects into a healthy and balanced daily life.
—Shakti Gawain

Stress is not all bad: We need stress hormones to get us out of bed in the morning and kick-start us into action. Our response to stress inspires us to organize our resources and take action when we have urgent action to take, like when you momentarily doze off while driving, drift into oncoming traffic, and are suddenly awakened by loud honking. Your stress response allows you to swerve and avoid the fatal collision.

The German philosopher Nietzsche said, "Whatever doesn't kill you makes you stronger." So, you become stronger and more resilient to stress when you are exposed to it. The damage results when stress is prolonged and without relief.

The physiological response of stress is a faster heartbeat, increased blood pressure, rising blood sugar levels, blood clot formation, disrupted digestion, and rerouting of blood to the extremities. It all depends on how you react to the stress. If you deal with it in a negative manner or it is prolonged, then you will become vulnerable to stress-related illnesses and shorten your life-span. Holistic health practitioner Paul Chek says: "Chronic stressors cause elevated stress hormones in the body, leading to immune system suppression, the inability to heal, and eventually to disease."

Health Miracle

Several studies have come to the same conclusion: Exercisers are less anxious, less depressed, less prone to anger, and more likely to have a good social network.

Fight or Flight

Up to 90 percent of doctor's visits may be triggered by a stress-related illness.
—The Center for Disease Control and Prevention in Atlanta

Our primitive ancestors used the fight-or-flight stress response for survival. But in modern times, this primal response is regularly activated by less than deadly situations (e.g., getting caught in a traffic jam, waiting to disembark from a plane, getting cut off in the buffet line—the list is infinite). In primitive times, fighting or fleeing relieved the stress. This doesn't work too well at the airport ticket counter!

Your body responds to an emergency by activating the sympathetic (fight-or-flight) nervous system, which sends out hormones like cortisol, epinephrine and norepinephrine and prepares your body for action by increasing the breathing rate, heart rate, blood pressure, and tensing muscles so you are ready to fight or flee. This is a completely healthy response, but it becomes very unhealthy when it is prolonged and results in elevated cortisol levels. Dr. Andrew Weil, author of *Healthy Aging*, says that cortisol "is directly toxic to neurons in the part of the brain that is responsible for memory and emotion." Some warning signs that your sympathetic nervous system might be overloaded are poor digestion, dry mouth, constipation, tension headaches, increased inflammatory conditions, problems with reproduction, anxiety, increased heart rate, feelings of being overwhelmed, and increased susceptibility to infection.

It doesn't end there. Dr. Len Kravitz, from the University of New Mexico, reports: "High levels of cortisol cause fat to be relocated and deposited deep in the abdomen, which left unchecked can develop into or enhance obesity." Deep abdominal fat, also known as central obesity, has been linked to type 2 diabetes, cerebrovascular disease, and cardiovascular disease. This deep abdominal fat can't be removed by plastic surgery; liposuction only takes away subcutaneous fat.

The potent stress hormone cortisol has also been implicated in the breakdown of muscle tissue. For a person who wants to look and feel youthful for a lifetime, this is very important to avoid. Research published in the *Journal of the American Geriatric Society* showed that loss of lean muscle mass is one of the central factors in premature aging.

Do You Have "Hurry Sickness?"

There is more to life than increasing its speed.
   —Gandhi

It's a 24-hour world. Are you in the rat race? If you are, you might want to consider what Lily Tomlin said: "Even if you win the rat race, you are still a rat." Between career demands, family events, voice mail, e-mail, text messages, conference calls, 900 channels on your television, and preparing your next meal, you barely have time to sleep! From the time you were a child, you were coached to look ahead, to plan for every possible event. At some point, you were probably even told to prebook your cemetery plot! Feeling "stressed" has become a way of life in the Western world.

As humans, not only do we deal with our everyday reality, we also deal with our unique ability to anticipate, remember, and visualize stress. Those of us who spend much of our days worrying about tomorrow or remembering what went wrong yesterday are continually experiencing the effects of chronic stress and anxiety.

Eckhart Tolle, the best-selling author of *The Power of Now*, says, "I have little use for the past and rarely think about it." Deepak Chopra speaks of the fact that many people are prisoners of their past, and that they need to spend more time focused on the present moment. In his book *Happiness Is a Choice*, Barry Neil Kaufman says, "People spend years, even lifetimes, rummaging through old memories and philosophies . . . we have to look forward toward a new vision that we can create—not merely in our lifetime, but right now."

> ### *Health Miracle*
>
> **Some of the prolific thinkers and writers in the field of personal development proclaim the wondrous effects of present moment focus. Living in the present provides a positive environment for personal happiness and peace of mind.**

Stress Can Make You Sick

We live in the midst of alarms; anxiety beclouds the future; we expect some new disaster with each newspaper we read.
   —Abraham Lincoln

Your nervous system is designed for action and resolution. It is not set up for extended periods of tension and insecurity. If you experience high levels of stress for a long enough period, you become vulnerable to mental illness. Depression, for example, is rampant in modern times. It is the number-one cause of disability in North America, according to the World Health Organization. One estimate is that depression due to stress will be so high by the year 2020 that only heart disease will affect more people.

Stress can also make you physically ill. We are sure at some point in your life you have worried about something for such a long time that you gave yourself a headache or stomach upset. But can stress actually give you a disease? According to Dr. Mary O'Brien, "Medical researchers and physicians are often hesitant to proclaim stress a risk factor for serious illness," and "at least so far, [it is] impossible to quantify."

Maybe stress doesn't directly cause disease, but it can provide a physiological environment that promotes disease. Some well-known studies like the Northwick Park Heart Study and the Framingham Study have shown anxiety to be a big risk factor in heart disease for men and women.

> **Health Miracle**
>
> In 1999, researchers at Duke University concluded that exercise was as effective as the antidepressant Zoloft.

Relaxation Response

The damage of chronic stress comes from your body's learned response to a situation—not from the situation itself. Learn ways to control your reactions to stressful situations.
—Eve Lees

Luckily, the body can affect the mind and we do have the ability to turn on a relaxation response in the body or shift from sympathetic (fight or flight) to parasympathetic nervous system dominance. When this happens, our metabolism and immunity function optimally: the heart rate slows, blood pressure falls, circulation is balanced, and digestive organs work smoothly. The parasympathetic system helps us achieve a state of calm or relaxation. This sounds like an ideal state to be in, doesn't it?

The rest of this chapter is a compilation of the top strategies you can utilize to activate your parasympathetic nervous system and reap the benefits of a newfound sense of well-being. Get ready for some phone calls—people who feel well are more fun to be around!

Stress Busters and Balance Boosters

If you want to minimize age-related deficits in mental function, you must know and practice strategies for neutralizing the harmful effects of stress on the brain and other organs.
—Dr. Andrew Weil

Deep Breathing

Breath is the stuff of life. If you have ever witnessed the miraculous birth of a baby, you have seen firsthand the human instinct to breathe. We start the human journey with an in-breath, and we end it with an out-breath.

At 12–15 times a minute, we breathe approximately 20,000 times a day. If you have poor posture or shallow breathing, your body will always feel like it isn't getting enough oxygen for its trillions of cells. If your body is struggling for its most basic needs, it might just be in a fight-or-flight mode most of the time. The result? A body that has a compromised immune system ages much more rapidly.

Breath is the number-one way to change your state and relax your nervous system. Anytime you take a deep breath, you are telling your brain that you are okay and relaxed. This is one of the easiest and fastest ways to elicit a relaxation response in the body. Just by practising a few minutes of deep, diaphragmatic breathing you can slow the heart, lower blood pressure, and reduce anxiety. You will also allow more oxygen to be carried to all the cells of the body, including the brain.

Cells cannot metabolize food properly without sufficient oxygen.

To begin, try breathing through your nose if you are able to. Your nose is lined with small hairs (cilia), which help to filter the air and remove impurities as they pass through the nasal canal. Also, the path to the lungs via the nose is longer and this allows the air to be warmed before it enters the delicate lung tissue. Lungs require a moist, warm environment for effective function.

Now make sure that you are seated comfortably, with good posture. Most office jobs lead to poor posture as the worker sits hunched in front of the computer. This leads to shallow breathing. So uncross your legs, disperse your weight evenly among your pelvic bones, and arch your lower back slightly so that your tailbone is pushed toward the back of your chair. Now align your shoulders and open your chest. You can achieve the correct upper body posture by raising your shoulders up toward your ears, then circling them back and down. You may need to repeat this a few times. You also need to center your head properly: push your chin back slightly so that you feel your head resting on top of your spine, centered between your shoulders. Now you are ready to breathe deeply.

Inhale slowly through your nose (if possible), allowing your abdomen to relax and expand. The relaxation of the abdomen allows the diaphragm (breathing muscle) to move downwards, which helps to draw oxygen deep into the lower lungs. Think of filling your lungs with oxygen like you would fill a barrel with water. Now exhale slowly, releasing the carbon dioxide from the top to the bottom of the lungs. You can squeeze the last bit of carbon dioxide from your lungs by gently engaging the abdominal muscles near the end of your exhale (draw the belly button in toward the spine). Try making your exhale as long as your inhale. (Inhaling and exhaling on a count of four works well. You can increase this number as your breathing skills improve.)

Take a Regular Time-out

Having regular time-outs are important to living a fully functioning life. The physical and mental benefits are numerous: better rest and relaxation, a feeling of balance, increased well-being through elevated levels of the feel good chemical serotonin, increased immune-system function, and lowered resting heart rate. There is nothing like a little solitude and quiet time to rejuvenate yourself.

Looking back or reflecting can be a great investment in your future. You can gather the lessons from your past and invest them in your next year. Remember it is your past, you have free license to rewrite some of the script. Wayne Dyer once said, "It is never to late to have a happy childhood."

So instead of living each year flying by the seat of your pants, you can move with more elegance and certainty into the future. As a result, you may become a better mother, a better father, a better spouse, a better friend, a better worker, or a better athlete. Try spending a few minutes each day looking back on the various lessons you've learned. Aim to set aside a special place in your house where you can collect your thoughts or just "be." You could decorate and paint a room so that it supports you emotionally and physically. It could be as simple as a comfortable chair in a quiet corner. Remember, the purpose of this activity is to focus on the growth and learning points you have gathered, and how they can be applied to the future. Don't fret about past mistakes or stresses. Just be open to the messages contained within your experiences.

Sleep

A good laugh and a long sleep are the best cures in the doctor's book.
—Irish proverb

A very good indicator of excellent mental and physical health is the ability to sleep soundly. Anxiety and stress can make a good night's sleep absolutely impossible, and not sleeping properly can lead to being stressed, so you can see how a vicious cycle can easily develop. A sound sleep, on the other hand, enables you to handle life's challenges and stressful events. Having a productive day starts with waking up refreshed and rejuvenated from a wonderful night's sleep.

The fact that millions of North Americans are taking sleep aids is an indicator that many of us aren't getting the quality shut-eye we would love. And if that is the case, you are starting the day behind the eight ball and it is virtually impossible to catch up.

Can a lack of sleep make you fat? Yes, it can. This little-known fact is often left off the list of things you can do to get leaner and healthier. Sleep experts recommend that people get a minimum of seven quality hours of sleep per night. Some people need eight or more. Dr. Deepak Chopra, author of over 50 books, says that the natural human sleep cycle is from 10 p.m. to 6 a.m.

The hormone that is a key player in your nighttime drama is melatonin. This all-important hormone is made in the pineal gland and in sufficient amounts it helps regulate sleep, blood pressure, sexual desire, menstruation, immune function, and makes your body more stress resistant. With respect to its effects on lean body mass, melatonin helps support growth hormone. Good levels of growth hormone mean you have great energy and a toned, supple body. Melatonin levels decline naturally as we age, so it becomes crucial to set the tone for a good night's rest. Feel like getting some ZZZZs? Here are our secrets for sound sleep:

1. Keep your bedroom cool, dark, and quiet for optimal sound sleep. This means no night-lights, or flimsy curtains that allow light into the room, disrupting the production of melatonin.

2. Create an evening routine that helps you wind down from your busy day. Dim the lights, refrain from intense mental or physical work, and use soft music to change your state. Try journaling, yoga, or meditation.

3. Refrain from drinking fluids before bedtime to avoid night time awakening for bathroom breaks.

4. Drinking alcohol may relax you to some extent, but the depth of sleep will not be as profound. The insulin spike from the alcohol and the resultant blood sugar drop could cause you to awaken during the night to eat because you will be hungry.

5. Keep caffeine to a minimum in the latter half of the day. Caffeine can take up to nine hours to be eliminated from your system and may linger until bedtime and disrupt your sleep.

6. Don't eat a large meal in the three hours before bedtime. Sleep is the time when our immune systems and repair systems function at their peak. This is the time for the body to clear up the waste of the day and repair any damage. If your body is busy digesting food while you sleep, it will be unable to perform its restorative work and the cycle of waking up tired continues!

The Odiatus' Story

We reached a crisis point around the time of our medically fragile son's third birthday. Since his birth, we had made a commitment

(continued)

to keep him at home with us. Jordan required frequent monitoring throughout the nights to ensure that he was positioned properly for clear breathing and to avoid choking on his own reflux. Three years of fractured sleep had taken its toll on us. Jordan's medical team at the hospital had warned us about this when he was born.

Depression started to sink its teeth into our family. Even though we are normally happy, healthy, optimistic people, we could not deny the physical and emotional effects our situation and lack of sleep were having on our health and wellness. It expressed itself in many forms: shingles, eczema, frequent colds, headaches, forgetfulness, short tempers, and a lack of concentration.

We used to think that our belief in God, our commitment to exercise, and our optimal nutrition could fix anything, but without adequate sleep over three years, even a gentle workout was painful. For the first time the gym provided no respite.

We loved our son dearly, but clearly needed some relief if we were to salvage our family and be able to care for him and his 14-month-old sister. Jordan transitioned into an amazing group home where a loving staff provides the 24-hour supervision and care that he requires. Since then, we have been able to get the sleep that we now know is essential to health, and we have reclaimed the energy to be able to shower our children with love.

Health Miracle

The Canadian Fitness and Lifestyle Research Institute reports that people who perform aerobic exercise regularly have an easier time falling asleep and are more likely to enter stage four sleep—the deep, restorative stage of sleep.

Massage

Also known as healing touch, massage is great for releasing tension and stress from the body. Just the act of being physically touched by another human being who has the intent to heal can potentially restore you to health. With a doctor's prescription, massage therapy is covered under most health insurance plans. Aim for a professional massage once per month. If your significant other is willing, why not take a partner massage course so that you can bond between professional treatments.

Progressive Muscle Relaxation

This is an easy form of relaxation that just requires a quiet place to sit or lie down. It is extremely helpful for sleep if you perform this as you lie in bed. Start with a natural deep-breathing rhythm. Then for a count of 10, contract all the muscles in your body. Clench your fists, flex your feet and toes, and tighten the muscles in your arms, legs, and face. Relax your body, letting the tension slowly release. Relax and breathe for about 30 seconds, then repeat two or three more times using a little less tension each time. You can also perform this by tensing and squeezing one part of the body at a time, moving from the feet all the way up to the face as you go.

Nutrition for Stress Relief

Certain foods like whole-grain carbohydrates stimulate serotonin production and are rich in B-vitamins, which help you deal with stress. Stress can deplete certain nutrients—vitamin C, iron, and calcium, for example. If you have a demanding life and experience a lot of stress, nutritious food choices are a must, and supplementation may be appropriate. Foods containing omega-3s have the ability to lower blood pressure, make platelets less sticky, and decrease fats in the blood, effectively lowering your risk for stroke and heart disease. As we have discussed in earlier chapters, dehydration and skipping breakfast are stressful to your body. Without a well-balanced meal in the morning, you will not have sufficient energy and nutrients to meet the demands of a busy day. And water is essential for all biochemical reactions in the body (thermoregulation, digestion, joint movement, waste and toxin removal), so make sure you get enough of it. Drink more if you are very active and during the heat of summer.

Try Color Breathing!

Some Chinese healers report that visualizing the colors of the spectrum can encourage relaxation and bring you peace. Research has shown that color affects you emotionally and physically. Chinese color therapists say that by first taking a deep breath and clearing your mind, you can then imagine breathing in a color and letting it flood your body. For example, it is believed that breathing in the color green—the color of nature—may stimulate the part of the nervous system that relaxes the muscles in your chest and helps you breathe more slowly.

Exercise

Exercise is nature's antidote to stress, anger, and frustration. Some therapists include walking as part of their clients' anger-management programs. Without regular activity, stress will linger in your system and take its toll on your body. Exercise can combat these negative effects by increasing neurotransmitters, neurotrophins, and connectivity in the brain. Throw in all the other benefits of exercise, such as self-confidence, improved appearance, and feeling younger and it's no wonder physical activity is the perfect remedy to stress!

Health Miracle

In Britain, doctors now use exercise as a first-line treatment for depression.

Qigong

Like tai chi, qigong (pronounced chi-gong) is a traditional Chinese exercise sequence that promotes increased energy flow and improved health through gentle, graceful, repeated movements. Proper breathing is an integral component of qigong, which is great for relieving stress and bolstering immunity. Qigong has been shown to improve posture, balance, coordination, endurance, and flexibility. Some participants experience a lowering of blood pressure.

Yoga

This ancient Hindu tradition helps you to tune in with your body. This body awareness can lead to better management of stress and food cravings. Yoga combines movement with breathing, and some classes will include exercises in meditation as well, so it is an excellent way to reap many benefits all at once. The increased sense of well-being provided by yoga gives you more tools to manage your emotions; it also gives you the benefits of increased flexibility, balance, and strength.

Uche's Story

It wasn't long ago that I used to have ongoing lower back pain. I had never included flexibility training in my workouts and I wasn't even close to being able to touch my toes. Each morning I would hear my alarm clock go off and struggle out of bed like an ornery bear. With my lower back tight and bladder full, I would lumber to the wash-room. One day I looked down and noticed my two cairn terriers going through their morning ritual of stretching. I couldn't help but think that these two canines didn't have any certification and did not know the Surgeon General's exercise recommendations!

"That's enough!" I thought to myself. The next day, I got down on all fours and imitated my furry pets. They seemed to take great plea-sure in watching me struggle with my stretches. Well, I got up, walked away with ease, and felt great the rest of the morning! The ripple ef-fect? I started going to yoga 90 minutes a week and began taking 10 minutes each morning to stretch and collect my thoughts. Today, I am pain-free and can easily touch my toes. Our massage therapist reports that my muscles feel smooth and pliable.

Quiet Time

Background noise is an enemy of healthy aging. We are plagued with the constant roar of automobiles, television, radio, air conditioning units, video games, aircraft, dogs barking—you name it. They all in-terfere with your homeostasis. The importance of peace and quiet is not a new notion. Philosophers and mystics throughout time have valued silence. In the Bible, Isaiah 26:20 says: "Come, my people, en-ter into your rooms and close your doors behind you; Hide for a little while until indignation runs its course." Scheduled quiet time will do wonders for your psyche. It will reduce stress and increase your energy.

Health Miracle

Peace of mind is a by-product of regular exercise. When you're doing something positive for your health, it's hard to focus on negative thoughts and feelings. Experts in the field of motiva-tion say it's psychologically impossible for your mind to hold two opposing thoughts in the same instant. Exercise can also give you a feeling of accomplishment and a sense of control, even if the rest of your life feels out of control.

Humor As a Healer

*Gladness of the heart is the life of a man and the joyfulness of a man prolon-
geth his days.*
  —Ecclesiastes 30:22

There are numerous studies on the benefits of laughter. William Fry,
M.D., author of numerous papers on the benefits of laughter, con-
tends that an extended session of laughter is equivalent to a session
of exercise. Stacks of research show there's a connection between
laughter and immune system enhancement. Laughter has also been
shown to have a positive impact on the muscular system, the central
nervous system, the respiratory system, the cardiovascular system, and
the endocrine system. And it appears to be one of the best natural
defenses against depression! It's too bad you can't buy it at your local
pharmacy!

Should hospitals hire nurses or doctors who have a background in
stand-up comedy? That could be a little challenging. Perhaps the most
difficult part would be finding the insurance code for the hospital to
charge for those services.

Dr. Norman Cousins, best-selling author of *Anatomy of an Illness*,
had an interesting story. He was a hard-working, popular professor at
the school of medicine at UCLA. Later in his career, he was confined
to a hospital bed with an aggressive connective-tissue disorder that limited his mobility. It caused extreme inflammation of his joints and spine
and put him in great pain.

Dr. Cousins asked a friend to set up a movie screen so he could
watch the Marx Brothers' movies and "Candid Camera" reruns all day.
When he found that 10 minutes of belly laughter gave him two hours
without pain, he knew he was onto something! Even his doctors noticed
that their patient looked better and needed a lot less pain medication
than they had been giving him. Laughter not only triggers endorphins,
the body's natural painkillers, it also increases the levels of serotonin,
one of the hormones connected with our sense of peace and security.
With the positive effects of his own special humor therapy, Dr. Cousins
eventually recovered most of his mobility.

Wilfred Peterson, author of *The Art of Living*, also recommends
laughter as a healing force. He noted that laughter sets healing vibrations

into motion and can fill any room with the sunshine of good cheer. Laughter can soothe a tense situation, calm a temper, and undo frazzled nerves. He said a daily prescription of "Don't take yourself so damned seriously" would work wonders for all of us.

> *He who laughs . . .*
> *lasts!*

Health Miracle

Laughter improves respiration and gently raises pulse and blood pressure before generating a relaxed state. It takes 43 muscles to frown versus only 17 to smile.

Incorporate Laughter into Your Day

Your brain produces a chemical that relays the news of your happiness to all of your body's cells—who rejoice and join in.
—Dr. Deepak Chopra

The love doctor Leo Buscaglia recommends that adults get in touch with their *kookiness* again. He reports that people take themselves too seriously and that bursts of laughter decrease as we age. He suggests living a little "nutty" occasionally. That alone can brighten any dreary day. Did you know that sharing funny stories and laughter with the important people in your life could strengthen the bond of your relationships? When you regularly laugh with your loved ones (not *at them*!), you begin associating good feelings with their presence.

Our wish for you is a life full of laughter and all of the health and soulful benefits that come with it! Laughter opens your heart and massages the soul. Start massaging today!

Happiness Homework

I realize that a sense of humor isn't for everyone. It's only for people who want to have fun, enjoy life, and feel alive.
—Anne Wilson Schaef

- Go to a comedy club with friends or your significant other on a regular basis.

- Go to your local bookstore and browse through the humor section—take a friend if you don't like laughing alone!

- Write down a list of activities in your journal that could bring more light and laughter to your life. Show this list to someone who might want to join you.

- Rent funny movies with some of your most outrageous friends.

- Go to the zoo during mating season. This is guaranteed to bring a smile to your face.

Being Present

The secret of health for both mind and body is not to mourn for the past, worry about the future, or anticipate troubles, but to live in the present moment wisely and earnestly.
—Buddha

No matter where you are or what you are doing, try to really be present. If you are with your children, give them your undivided attention; don't worry about work or next week. If you are working, do your best, even if you are not at your dream job. If you have a long commute to work, find positive ways to spend this time (like listening to peaceful music or audiobooks) instead of cursing at the traffic.

Life is all about experiences—some are good, some are not so good. Part of growth is that there will be some risks and challenges along the way. That is the teeter-totter of life, so instead of searching for some ideal, we need to create our own healthy existence by preparing ourselves for the ups and the downs. We can't change the stresses in our world, but we do have control over how we perceive the stresses and how we deal with them. This will lead to a sense of well-being, which may be the closest we come to being in balance.

Health Miracle Activities

1. Is there an area of your life that you need to simplify?

_____

_____

2. Is there a place in your life where there is unfinished business?

_____

_____

3. What action step can you take to move toward a resolution today?

_____

_____

4. What stress-busting strategy will you begin with?

_____

_____

Chapter 12

It's lack of faith that makes people afraid of meeting challenges, and I believed in myself.
  —Muhammad Ali

Spiritual Fitness

To be alive is to be moving.
Inhibit the movement and you create illness.
To block movement is to block change.
The moving body freely channels the energy of life.
        —John Travis and Regina Sara Ryan

Everyone has a spiritual side or a yearning to find meaning and purpose in life. It doesn't really matter how you practise your spirituality—just know that it is vital for you to make time to be alone with your thoughts on a regular basis. Dr. Kenneth R. Pelletier believes that the characteristics of spirituality are "eminently conducive to health and well-being." In his book, *The Best Alternative Medicine*, he describes spirituality as "an inner sense of something greater than oneself, recognition of a meaning to existence."

Our spirit connects us to our values and this will have an impact on the choices we make about food and exercise. Spirituality has been a part of healing since the beginning of human history, yet only recently have modern-day scientists agreed that ancient healing techniques are worthy of consideration and study.

Have you ever thought that there was more to you than your body? That there's a part of you that is unchanging and is the true essence of who you are? There is more to becoming healthy and fit than just having a flat stomach, toned arms, and buns of steel. There is spiritual fitness. It refers to the level of harmony between body, mind, and spirit.

Wayne Dyer, in *Your Sacred Self*, explains that we grow up believing we are a body, a job, or a nationality. We encourage you to break free from these physical descriptions. It's an established scientific fact that every seven years, the cells in your body will have been replaced with new cells. This means your physical self is constantly changing. In other words, eight years ago, your body was composed of totally different cells than it is today! What part of you is responsible for the memories and feelings from eight or more years ago? The essence of what makes you an individual is beyond the physical—it is timeless, ageless, and without form. As Marianne Williamson says, "We can be physically older but emotionally and psychologically younger." Our bodies may age, but our spirit does not.

Health Miracle

The U.S. National Institute for Healthcare Research has found many studies in which participation in religious activities offered protection against immune dysfunction, heart disease, depression, anxiety, and suicide.

The People of Okinawa

Training gives us an outlet for suppressed energies created by stress and thus tones the spirit just as exercise conditions the body.
    —Arnold Schwarzenegger

Earlier in the book we spoke of the Okinawans' way of eating, but that is not the only component that contributes to their amazing health and longevity. Exercise is a way of life there. The Okinawans are fit in all three components of fitness: strength, flexibility, and aerobic. Even more interesting is the Okinawans' philosophy that exercise is connected with their spirituality. Their belief is that nurturing life energy and living in balance with nature will garner health and longevity. Martial arts, traditional dance, gardening, and walking all form the base of the Okinawan mind-body fitness program.

Exercise As a Path

Do not neglect this body. This is the house of God; take care of it, only in this body can God be realized.
    —Nisargadatta Maharaj

In *Working Out, Working Within,* Jerry Lynch and Chungliang Al Huang reveal that there is increased creativity and mental clarity with the "stillness in motion" achieved during exercise. Because exercise needs such intense focus and concentration, you have the opportunity to transcend your day-to-day challenges. Some people call this "the zone."

We both love the gym for many reasons other than for its calorie-burning qualities. We have connected our time in the gym to physical and mental relief. There's really nothing quite like a good workout and its ability to change your emotional state. Frustration, anxiety, fear, sadness, anger all get washed away when you exercise.

So, if you're challenged by something in your life, one of the best ways to get a handle on it is to get moving and enjoy some physical exertion. Through exercising, you may access a wellspring of knowledge and inner creativity. Even going for a short walk can give you a chance to shed some light on a problem. Exercise might be the one thing you haven't tried to solve that ongoing personal challenge.

Kary's Story

I turn to exercise whenever I feel a need to connect with my higher self. Some of my greatest insights and "ah-ha's" have come to me during a long walk in nature, or in the middle of an intense cardio workout. The best part of my fitness program is the yoga and deep-breathing sequence that I perform at the end of every workout session. This is my time to find the "stillness in motion" that can rejuvenate my mind and spirit as well as my body.

Health Miracle

Nike, HBO, Forbes, and Apple all offer on-site yoga classes for their employees. These and scores more Fortune 500 companies consider yoga important enough to offer classes as a regular employee benefit.

Meditate Your Way to Spiritual Fitness

In the final analysis, the hope of every person is peace of mind.
—Dalai Lama

> *People who meditate regularly experience a 50 percent lower cancer rate and an 80 percent lower heart disease rate!*

Jon Kabat-Zinn's book, *Wherever You Go, There You Are,* defines meditation as a way of being, living, and listening, a way of being in harmony with things as they are.

Enjoying a reflective component in our daily lives may be essential to happiness and peace of mind, but how many of us are making time for it? Perhaps we should take the hint from enlightened teachers like: Jesus, Buddha, Mohammad, Shankara, Lao Tzu, and Mother Teresa who have acknowledged that an inner journey is essential for peace and happiness.

Many people have the misconception that the only way to meditate is to sit in the lotus position with a candle and some crystals by your side, but there are numerous meditative strategies stemming from different religions and philosophies. Meditation doesn't have to be a complicated process. It can be as simple as closing your eyes and taking some deep breaths before you leave for work—try the deep-breathing exercise from the previous chapter.

It can be as simple as enjoying the sound of water falling over rocks or the air passing through your nostrils into your lungs. During meditation, your mind has a sense of clarity, of being free from the stress of self-consciousness. Time is unimportant and seems to fly by. These are moments when you are carefree and joyful; these are moments of flow that can occur anytime, anywhere.

The next time you are feeling a little down, take a time-out and turn inward. Instead of turning on the television, reading a magazine, or going to the refrigerator, get comfortable in a chair or on the floor. Just sit down and take some deep breaths, if only for a minute or two. Simply sit and be still. See if you are able to recapture some energy and vitality.

You will be in good company if you start the practice of meditation: spiritual sages throughout history have spent a part of their day in silence or meditation. Adding this regular discipline to your schedule would provide an opportunity for you to review your day and make daily adjustments for tomorrow. Denying yourself time for your soulful, boundless, spiritual side is like chopping down trees, day after day, without ever sharpening your ax.

We've read that 4:00 a.m. is a great time to awaken and be alone with your thoughts. Spiritual teachers have long heralded this time of day as a magical time to tap into consciousness. It is a special time when we're not bothered by distractions, like the telephone or the noise of traffic. Obviously it would take a fair amount of discipline to begin the practice of rising at 4:00 am., so maybe start with a few minutes of reflection upon rising in the morning. Robin Sharma, author of *The Monk Who Sold His Ferrari*, reported that reflection and journaling are a big part of his success.

Uche's Story

I graduated from university with a wealth of technical and clinical information. I could do extremely challenging dental procedures and recite facts to back up any point of view. I was able to work a full 10-hour day and go to the gym—without a break. I felt invincible at the age of 28.

One day my brother, Chiedu, gave me inspirational speaker Les Brown's video called Live Your Dreams. *I became fascinated with the topic of what made human beings tick. I began to take workshops in my city. I became adventurous and invested in conferences outside my city (and later the country). I had the opportunity to meet and learn from some amazing people at the forefront of personal development and spirituality. I enrolled in courses on meditation, self-development, and communication. The list was endless.*

I felt I was really beginning to get a grasp on the entire subject. But it always brings a smile to my face when I remember a telephone conversation with my mother. I was trying to explain some challenge I was facing. I told her I was about to try one of the new strategies I had learned at an expensive three-day, professional lecture series. She replied, "That's a lot of money to spend, son. Have you tried praying yet?"

Health Miracle

According to researchers from the Stress Reduction Clinic at the University of Massachussetts Medical Center in Worcester, yoga, in conjunction with meditation, can indeed relieve stress and improve work performance. The Stress Reduction Clinic is the oldest and largest hospital-based mind-body center of its kind in the U.S. It has treated more than 10,000 patients since opening in 1979.

The Miracle of Practising Forgiveness

I can't think of any disease that ages a person faster than chronic anger and resentment.
   —Mary O'Brien, M.D.

So many people carry their wounds and grudges around like a ball and chain—no, you can't count this as a resistance training workout!—that drag you down and hold you back from personal joy and growth. This is important on a physical and psychological level. Anger and resentment are two of the most destructive emotions a person can feel. We are not saying that you have to ask the perpetrator of your wounds back into your life, but you must learn to forgive and forget in order to protect your own health.

Spiritual lecturer and author Marianne Williamson says that we must let go of our condemnation, not only to free someone else, but to free ourselves as well. This can be accomplished by looking beyond the physical nature of the person who has hurt us. Look instead to his or her soul and believe that there is innocence inside, and allow yourself to release the weight of your condemnation. Confucius said, "To be wronged is nothing unless you continue to remember it." The only thing worth remembering is the lesson you have learned. Every experience in life, bad or good, contains a lesson if you are willing to look for it.

Health Miracle

Studies have associated forgiveness with lower heart rate, blood pressure, and stress relief.

Alter Your Physical Reality

Nothing in life is more wonderful than faith—the one great moving force that we can neither weigh in the balance nor test in the crucible.
   —Sir William Osler

By working to achieve inner harmony, you can alter your physical reality. Every one of the 120 trillion cells in your body is affected by your thoughts and feelings. Each of those cells is eavesdropping on our inner and outer dialogue. Candace Pert, Ph.D., in her groundbreaking book, *Molecules of Emotion*, tells how our thoughts and feelings have far-ranging effects on our physical selves: "the body is the outward manifestation of the mind."

Christiane Northrup, M.D., author of *Mother-Daughter Wisdom*, acknowledges that consciousness affects everything you do. We need to acknowledge this connection, and if we don't, we can find ourselves caught up in a spiral of aches, pains, and medications. To begin healing, we must first take responsibility for the condition we are in. If we are at the top of the list for causes of the pain, then we can be at the top of the list for solutions.

Louise Hay, metaphysical lecturer and best-selling author of over 20 books, is a strong believer in the power of listening to our bodies for healing. She says that if we take the time to be silent and to look inward, we are able to truly listen to what our bodies are saying. In *You Can Heal Your Life*, she explains how the different physical ailments that plague us are mostly caused by toxic thoughts and emotions. We will go deeper into this subject in our next chapter: "Health and the Law of Attraction."

Seven Spiritual Habits of Health

It is a happy talent to know how to play.
—Emerson

1. **Spend some time in nature.** This could mean taking yourself and your loved ones on a day trip into nature. For example, hiking on a mountain trail, a picnic on an isolated beach, or a trip to the lake. Away from the incessant demands of work and the city, you have the opportunity to get in touch with yourself. There's nothing more refreshing than breathing fresh air and marveling at the beauty of nature in all her glory! We were moved when we read James Redfield's book *Celestine Vision: Living the New Spiritual Awareness*. He writes of special spots and mystical sites on the planet—the great pyramids, Stonehenge, and many others. You can visit these places or find your own special spots that give you a sense of well-being, rejuvenation, and energy.

2. **Spend some time in an art gallery or museum.** The appreciation of art can momentarily assist you in transcending daily challenges. Throughout history art has played a role in raising consciousness. In the Golden Age of Greece, it was statues. Before the Renaissance, suppressed scholars in Europe sought intellectual and spiritual

rejuvenation through painting. When can you make time to visit a gallery and tap into this energy? You may not be able to get to Paris today, but every major city and many smaller towns have an art gallery or museum.

3. **Get up for the sunrise or plan an evening walk during sunset.** In ancient times, spending time in the sun was thought to connect us with our souls. People would worship the sun for all the gifts it brought them. Research shows that sun exposure is important for the production of vitamin D in the body.

4. **Create a sacred space.** A special spot reserved just for your spiritual fitness may seem like a luxury, but is well worth creating. Thomas Edison and Benjamin Franklin had an area set aside in their homes where they sat alone with their thoughts. Your spot could be located outside if you prefer. Dr. Deepak Chopra loves the idea of a natural sanctuary. He reports that it can increase your *Prana* or *Chi* (life force energy), which has the effect of replenishing or rejuvenating a tired spirit. There's power in silence. Without the silence between the notes, there would be no music! Silent contemplation can and will deliver many gifts for you. Not only will it make you stronger mentally and spiritually, it will have surprising effects on you physically.

5. **Read stimulating books.** Whenever you feed your mind, you have the opportunity to nourish your spirit. Books allow the curious person to tap into the treasure chest of others' experiences. The great French philosopher Rene Descartes said, "The reading of all good books is like a conversation with the finest minds of past centuries."

6. **Listen to music.** Have some instrumental CDs close at hand. Try any of Mozart's music, Vivaldi's *The Four Seasons*, or anything by Andrea Bocelli for starters. Soothing music can calm frazzled nerves at the end of a long day, especially if you get stuck in traffic on the way home from work. If you feel like sharing your enthusiasm for classical music, open up the sunroof. And if you are so moved to sing along with Andrea Bocelli, just keep your cell phone handy so you can pretend you are talking into it if someone happens to look over.

7. Look for the gift. There is always an equivalent benefit anytime you have a setback in your life. It may not become clear until many years later, but looking for the gift sooner will make your journey through life easier. For example, a man once lost his job. Instead of wallowing in self-pity, he saw his new free time as a gift. He joined a running club while searching for a new job. He met someone at the club who had an excellent business opportunity for him. His choice to make the most of his situation led to many payoffs: his physical health improved, he avoided depression, and he found a new job opportunity. Writer William Ernest Henley wrote "I am the master of my fate, I am the captain of my soul." By actually designing our response, we can be the architects of our destinies! Do not wish for fewer challenges; ask instead for more strength to handle the obstacles.

Health Miracle

The Durham Veterans Administration Hospital conducted a large study in 1988. They found less depression in men who relied on religious practices to cope during their hospital stays.

Health Miracle Activities

1. Do you have any people in your life who you would say are spiritually fit?

2. What spiritual practices do you have in your life?

3. Which spiritual practices would you be able to try in the next week?

Chapter 13

What is the definition of any miracle? Something that happens outside of convention, outside of the box that's socially acceptable, scientifically acceptable, religiously acceptable. And right outside the box is where human potential exists.

—Joe Disperza, D.C.

Health and the Law of Attraction

Imagination is everything. It is the preview of life's coming attractions.
    —Albert Einstein

There is a timeless, ageless phenomenon that has been referred to by sages, teachers and authors as the Law of Attraction, the Power of Intention, or *The Secret*. Hundreds of years ago, you may have been ridiculed or burnt at the stake for implying thoughts could become things. Today science would include the study of these powerful forces in quantum physics.

We won't delve too deeply into the mysteries of quantum physics, although we do recommend the book (or movie) called *What the Bleep Do We Know?!* to anyone who is interested in learning more about this intriguing and exciting area of study. In a nutshell, our thoughts do affect our world. People who have great health are thinking mostly thoughts of health and wellness, just as anyone with great wealth thinks mostly about abundance. Like attracts like—it is as simple as that.

Paul Pearsall, Ph.D., in *Making Miracles*, explained how events do not always happen separately from us, but rather, they are connected to our interpretations and actions. This can be an unsettling topic, but we urge you to suspend your current feelings and beliefs and read on.

Take a moment to do a quick inventory of your predominant thoughts about your health and your body. Don't worry if it's a little bleak, but understand that this may be your main block to tipping the scale in favor of abundant health and energy.

Dr. Joe Dispenza reports that "Your brain doesn't know the difference between what's taking place out there and what's taking place in here," so in this chapter we will encourage you to start changing your inner world in order to experience change in your physical world. Don't worry about how it will happen or when—just trust that when you start radiating what you desire from the inside, it will manifest in your life.

> ### Health Miracle
>
> **The body is designed to heal itself. There are countless reports of recoveries and of spontaneous remissions from disease.**

It's More than Luck

I am a great believer in luck, and I find the harder I work, the more I have of it.
  —Stephen Leacock

We believe "luck" and "chance" are overused words. For example, "I'm not sure how I won that race; I guess I was just lucky," or "Someday I'll get my chance." When life is lived intentionally—that is, when there are clearly defined goals and when your thoughts are in sync with your desires—you can see opportunities as they present themselves and take advantage of them. This is the Law of Attraction at work.

We challenge you to see yourself as having more control over the events in your life than you may have previously thought. Psychologist Carl Jung talked about chance events. He referred to coincidence as a bridge between science and spirit. In other words, there may be more than chance at play when you answer the phone and the person you were just thinking about happens to be on the other end. It's almost as if there is some divine plan with respect to the way events happen *coincidentally*. Albert Einstein said, "Coincidences are God's way of remaining anonymous." Hey, if you were 20 pounds overweight with high blood pressure and you sat down next to a personal trainer on an airplane, we would call that divine intervention!

Feel Your Way to Health

Every patient carries his or her own doctor inside.
   —Albert Schweitzer

If you are feeling horrible about the way you look and always thinking unproductive thoughts when it comes to your health, it's time to recognize it and release it immediately. Your results will often be in harmony with your thoughts. You probably know someone in your life who speaks about illness and disease constantly. Doesn't that person often seem to be sick?

It's time to stop telling yourself: "I was bad today, I cheated on my diet, I'm so fat. I want to lose weight, but I can't stop eating the damn chips." It doesn't matter if you are saying the words out loud or keeping them to yourself. They will have a negative effect on every cell in your body. It is one thing to hear another person put you down; it is even worse to be the one putting yourself down. You must strive to get over your own feelings of hopelessness and self-loathing, they are very destructive emotions. David Hawkins, M.D., Ph.D., author of *Power vs. Force*, stated that guilt and shame are two of the lowest energy states the human psyche can feel.

Change and the Law of Attraction

What things so ever ye desire, when ye pray, Believe that ye receive them, and ye shall have them.
   —Mark 11:24

Change is not easy—it's almost like every cell in our bodies resist it. "My life isn't that bad. It could be worse. At least I'm not as big as that lady down the street." Or at least that is what you have talked yourself into. And that's okay—maybe it's not your time for a new way of life. But if you are ready—if you have any feeling that there must be something more for you—then read on! All you need is someone to show you that your desires are possible. You need more information about putting the Law of Attraction to work and you need to embrace the knowledge that it is possible for you. Don't worry, you will put this information to use sooner or later. It doesn't matter when. Once you take that step and go for that something more, you will experience a profound sense of joy and personal satisfaction.

When you are feeling good about yourself, that is the time to really enjoy your feelings and thoughts. Breathe deeply and allow yourself to bask in these feelings, which will start the attraction process of more good feelings. Your thoughts have a remarkable impact on your actions and vice versa. If you don't treat yourself well, then you are saying that you're not deserving, or you're not good enough or important enough. And if you don't think well of yourself, it will be impossible to treat yourself with love and respect by eating nutritious foods and exercising your body.

Uche's Story

I was in my mid-thirties, a successful, single dentist, yet something was missing—and I was totally open to change. One day a receptionist in my office mentioned that her boyfriend was involved in Toastmasters. I had a flashback to a Grade 10 teacher telling me that I had a unique ability to engage people in what I was saying, so I called the receptionist's boyfriend and asked if I could join the next meeting.

I enjoyed it so much that I started attending courses on speaking, writing, and self-development. I began journaling and would often describe my ideal day, and my ideal soul mate. I often visualized myself speaking to large groups of people, but the topic was not clear.

I had been involved with the sport of bodybuilding since I was 14 years old. I competed provincially, nationally, and internationally while at dental school, and I became the president of the Manitoba Amateur Bodybuilding Association. My first speaking opportunity came when I found out that as president, I was expected to emcee the annual bodybuilding competitions. My co-emcee was Canadian Fitness Champion, Kary Larkin, who eventually became my wife. We were both passionate about health and it seemed natural to expand our emceeing into live seminars and a book.

Fast-forward 10 years and I am living the life I described so vividly in my journals—practising dentistry a few days a week, becoming a published author, marrying the woman of my dreams, and traveling all over the world to share the miracle of health with people.

Bridge the Gap

If you realized how powerful your thoughts are, you would never think a negative thought.
—Peace Pilgrim

Psychology states that you get what you focus on. Focused attention has the power to narrow the gap between the things you want in life and achieving them. Focused attention has organizing ability. It has the ability to make things happen. You must know someone who wanted something so badly, he or she worked at it by day and dreamed about it at night. It's almost as if they said, "Move over world, I'm coming through." Randy Pausch, in his best-seller *The Last Lecture*, said, "A lot of people want a shortcut. I find the best shortcut is the long way, which is basically two words: work hard."

You can apply this very effective tool to achieving more health for yourself or anything else for that matter. Simply focus your attention on what you want and resolve to see it through to completion. Don't fall for the quick-fix schemes and diet plans. Healthy, fit people do things a certain way, and they take daily action on a consistent basis.

One of the definitions of insanity is doing the same thing over and over and expecting a different result. Well, having the same outlook on health, exercise, nutrition, and wondering why you still hate your stomach or have had a bad back for what seems like months is tantamount to being insane. Nothing can change until you change the way you look at food, working out, and dieting. The solution is pretty simple.

Health Miracle

Eating shouldn't be so complicated. As a society, we have lost our intuitive relationship with food. We eat because it's time to eat, because food is placed in front of us, or because we are lonely—not because we are actually hungry. A study in the *New England Journal of Medicine* found that preschool children could intuitively regulate how much they ate according to their bodies' requirements for growth.

Possibility Thinking

There is a law in psychology that if you form a picture in your mind of what you would like to be, and you keep and you hold that picture there long enough, you will soon become exactly as you have been thinking.
—William James

Dr. Wayne Dyer tells a story about the first ships that were made out of materials other than wood. Nobody thought cast-iron ships would float. The flotation of cast-iron ships did not come about with the contemplation of the sinking of things! Just think of Columbus—his mind was not full of ideas of a flat planet when he headed out on his journey to prove that the world was round! The Wright brothers weren't dreaming about their plane staying on the ground! So, you won't get lean by obsessing about your stomach roll. Open your mind to a new way of looking and thinking about your body. Focus on what you want, not what you don't want. Focus on your ideal body shape and weight. Look for examples of people who have achieved the goals you desire. Open your mind to the possibility that you too can move in that direction.

The Power of Focus

Opportunities multiply as they are seized.
—Sun Tzu

Consider this: On a sunny day, every child on the playground feels the warmth of the sun, 93 million miles away. Yet a child with a magnifying glass can focus the sun's rays to "magically" burn a hole through a leaf. Similarly, you have the ability to tap into the amazing power of focus when you magnify the magical abilities of your mind. Anytime you take energy and concentrate it, you have the ability to make things happen. Efforts that are spread too thin rarely achieve anything.

If your goal is to live a life of health and vitality, you'll need to go about it with focused effort. It's not just going to happen on its own. Focused effort means you will be actively looking for information about fitness. You'll be asking questions of people who already have bridged the gap between *wanting* and *doing*. With this kind of energy and enthusiasm, you'll find yourself in the right place at the right time for going across the bridge. Things will start happening in your favor to move you closer to whatever it is you want. Did you know there is a physical part of your body (called the reticular activating system) that can be used to assist you in this process?

Reticular Activating System

Our body is really the product of our thoughts.
   —Dr. John Hagelin

Start saying the word "green" over and over to yourself and as you look around your environment, everything that is green will pop out at you. This is an example of the network of neurons in your brain called the reticular activating system (RAS) at work. Maxwell Maltz, in *Psycho-Cybernetics*, explains how the RAS acts like a heat-seeking missile whenever your interest is piqued.

For example, if you are becoming interested in your health, you may start noticing all the different types of food people eat. You may notice that there are three health-food stores on your drive home. Or if you are looking for a piece of home gym equipment, you may notice more advertisements on television for fitness-related products. You may also notice more people engaged in fitness activities. You may say to yourself, "Why are there so many people out jogging these days?"

Of course, new health-food stores aren't popping up all over your route home—it's just that your focused attention literally pulls things out of your environment and puts them at the forefront of your consciousness.

Remember when you were looking to buy a specific kind of car? And you spent all that time and energy on test-drives and then finally made the purchase? Remember after you bought it? It seemed like *everyone* was driving your make of car. You would see them everywhere. Your consciousness was highly charged. Your RAS was still on red alert.

This kind of *thought concentration* has many profound implications. It's like stoking a fire. *New York Times* best-selling author Paulo Coelho, in *The Alchemist*, describes the phenomenon of how the universe conspires to help anyone who focuses his or her intentions. Serendipitous occasions take place: someone gives you a health-related book as a gift;

your friend calls to ask if you want to go to a new yoga class; you find out your company has included physiotherapy in your benefits package. You may think it's luck or coincidence, but *no*, your intense focus and desire for health has attracted vehicles to take you closer to your goal.

Uche's Story

I had my car serviced and our mechanic casually asked me if we had ever thought of getting snow tires. I had never put much thought into it and I didn't even know what they looked like. He showed me a set and explained that they would increase traction in our harsh Canadian winter driving conditions. While driving later that day, I looked over at a car and noticed snow tires. I looked over a few times and thought to myself, "Hey, that person is really concerned about traction in snow. Maybe we should get some snow tires." After those few moments of attention, I moved on to other thoughts and finally got to my destination. For the next few days, I kept seeing cars with snow tires wherever I went! Out of the corner of my eye, while stopping to get gas, pulling up to park in a parking stall, there they were—snow tires!

To achieve what you want, be it health, success, great wealth, or recognition, you must want it strongly enough, with all of the might of your being, to achieve, to possess, or to be healed.
      —Howard Hill

Your Amazing Mind

Attracting the perfect weight is the same as placing an order with the catalogue of the Universe. You look through the catalogue, choose the perfect weight, place your order, and then it is delivered to you.
      —Rhonda Byrne

Your mind is divided into two parts: your conscious mind and your unconscious mind. The key thing for you to know about the conscious part of your mind is that you can choose your thoughts; you can actually communicate with your conscious mind directly through your self-talk. *New York Times* best-selling author James Ray, in *The Science of Success*, says: "The thoughts you choose create impulses of energy that vibrate all through your body and beyond and eventually determine your results in life." You have to stop ruminating about the roll on your stomach, your graying hair, and your aging body if you want to start moving toward wellness! The more you dwell on what you don't like about yourself, the more you will experience what you don't want. Eckhart Tolle in his *New York Times* best-seller *A New Earth* reports that you can't manifest what you want, only what you are. So begin now—hold your shoulders back like a healthy person with good posture, take an apple for a snack like an athlete would, and go for a walk like an active person would.

The *Course in Miracles* teaches that we give in to thoughts of self-deprecation and limitation because our minds are undisciplined. Your unconscious mind is listening to every thought you allow into your conscious mind. Your entire body responds to everything you say and think. Marianne Williamson says: "With every thought, you can start to re-create your life." It's time to lighten up your thoughts! Pardon the pun.

If you are a little unsure of this information, just know that the results you have achieved in your life to date have been obtained by your thoughts, feelings, and actions. If you are not happy with your results, then you need a new way of looking and feeling about health, wellness, and your vitality. Remember what theoretical physicist Albert Einstein said: "You can't solve a problem with the same mindset or consciousness that created it."

According to the Law of Attraction, you will manifest in your life all of the things you focus on, so by focusing attention on the things you don't like about yourself (i.e., excess weight), you will just attract more of those things to you! If you are currently unable to look in the mirror and honestly say that you like yourself—or, dare we go as far as to say, love yourself—we feel there is a need for a *thought makeover.* If you drag yourself to the gym because you can't bear to see yourself aging or gaining weight, we feel you are in need of a new way to look at exercise. Many philosophers have observed that people attract the very things they are afraid of.

Kary's Story

I used the Law of Attraction or Power of Intention or the Secret to achieve my ultimate dream of competing at the Fitness Olympia. I had been competing for almost 10 years and I was still nowhere near qualifying. You have to place top three in a professional fitness event in order to qualify for the Olympia. My best placing had been sixth place—in my own country! No one believed it was possible for me, and Uche and I wanted to start a family soon. I was 33 years old and I did not have the athletic background that most of the top pros did. Many of my competitors were former champion gymnasts, dancers, or cheerleaders. I was just a girl from a small town in Manitoba, Canada. Most people didn't even understand how I had made it to the professional ranks in the first place. But they underestimated the Power of Intention. You see, I had been reading about this concept years before the movie—The Secret—became popular.

Uche and I decided that I should take one last shot at the qualification. There was a pro show in Hungary coming up, and we agreed that if I didn't make it, we would throw in the towel and start our family. I started a daily meditation to clear my mind of all things negative and immediately afterward I would visualize the competition with a third place finish for me. I visualized myself on the stage, the emcee calling my name for third. I felt the joy of knowing that the years of my hard work and dedication were finally paying off.

The time came and we flew to Europe to prepare for the competition. On the day of the show I knew that I could not have done any more. I let go of all my angst and worry and decided to have the best show of my life because it might be my last. I gave up the need to place and I concentrated instead on the gratitude I felt for being able to live the last 10 years of my life as an athlete. I thought of all the joy competing had brought to me over the years and I really let go. To make a long story short, I got up on that stage and felt like I was on fire! Both of my routines were flawless and I was called out with the top girls for the physique judging. At the end of the night as I waited for the results, I felt a calm overtake me. It didn't really matter what happened. I then heard the magical words: "In third place, qualifying for the Olympia, Kary Odiatu from Canada!!!"

Tools of Intention

Life is like a combination lock; your job is to find the right numbers, in the right order, so you can have anything you want.
—Brian Tracy

Now that your mind is open to receiving, we urge you to read over the following tools of intention that we have compiled to assist you on the path to your own health miracles. Remember to release the need to know how or why you will get your results. Just trust in the Law of Attraction and utilize these powerful tools. The benefits will be out of this world!

Gratitude

When you feel grateful, you become great, and eventually attract great things.
—Plato

Success expert James Ray says that you need to know and live some basic truths about gratitude: you must appreciate the things you already have and believe that things will get better and better. We know gratitude is one of the highest emotional states that can bring some of the greatest rewards in your quest for health and wellness. In Wallace Wattles's *Secret of Getting Rich*, he has an entire chapter on gratitude. He wrote that it's very important to be thankful for what you have in the present moment. Approximately 150,000 people die each day according to the *Central Intelligence Agency World Factbook*. So you can be thankful that you are alive and reading this material right now. You have probably heard of the saying, "Any day above ground is a good day."

Our friend Sean Stephenson, who is the guy who wasn't supposed to live because of his debilitating brittle-bone condition, once told us that he woke up one day in his early teens and realized that he needed to stop feeling sorry for himself. After all, he was alive! And he started to focus on that gratitude. He turned his whole life around and used his condition as a platform for writing and speaking to thousands of teenagers about having *no excuses* in life. Sean has been on *Oprah* and he has even worked with President Bill Clinton. Barry Neil Kaufman, in *Happiness Is a Choice*, said, "If just one person changes, becomes happier, touches another with a more loving and peaceful hand, then the world has, indeed, become a more peaceful place."

> **Health Miracle**
>
> The international best-seller *The Secret* promises that just 30 days of filling yourself with gratitude will change your life.

Desire

Desire is the starting point of all achievement, not a hope, not a wish, but a keen pulsating desire which transcends everything.
   —Napoleon Hill

Wanting something to take place in your life is the seed of creation; it is the beginning of everything. Wayne Dyer, Ph.D., author of *Manifest Your Destiny*, reported that the universe has no waste. Everything in our world has a reason for existing, so every desire contains within it the necessary resources to make it a reality. If we dream of participating in a full marathon, then we are fully capable of doing so! We would not have the idea or inclination if it were not possible for us.

Feel

Be careful what you set your heart upon for it will surely be yours.
   —James Baldwin

Once you have a desire for your health, then you need to bring some emotion to the desire. Your feelings and emotions create a sense of urgency. It is necessary to fuel your desires with positive feelings and emotions. If you have a desire to have better flexibility and freedom of movement, then you need to feel what that will be like. Allow yourself to soak in your emotions as you visualize yourself moving with ease. Feel the joy and happiness that this would bring to you.

Visualization

See the things that you want as already yours. Know they will come to you at need. Then let them come. Don't fret and worry about them. Don't think about your lack of them. Think of them as yours, as belonging to you, as already in your possession.
   —Robert Collier

Robert J. Ringer, in *Million Dollar Habits*, depicted a positive correlation between what we visualize and the results we achieve. Having a clear mental image of our goals and dreams is vital to achieving them. Keeping your goals in mind and rehearsing the celebration of achievement are powerful tools that can keep you focused as you move forward. Mary Lou Retton, 1984 U.S. Olympic gymnastic gold medalist, mentally rehearsed a perfect gymnastics routine thousands of times before she actually achieved her dream. At first, this method seemed absurd to athletes who didn't understand how sitting still and closing their eyes could improve their performance. Today this exercise is common at all high levels of competition. Visualize your desire, and feel the emotions that would come with its achievement.

We like to visualize our goals, dreams, and desires in many ways. We have created a "vision board" on one side of our bedroom wall. It is a large corkboard that we have filled with images of things we would like to attract into our lives. Anything goes! We have pictures of our dreams and goals plastered all over it. We even have a map with pins on the cities we would like to visit. Our kids love the vision board—it is bright and colorful and we will help them create their own one day.

Health Miracle

Edmund Jacobson, M.D., discovered that the brain does not know the difference between a visualized action and a performed action. Close your eyes now and see yourself living the health and fitness lifestyle of your dreams.

Reflect

Each time you make a positive choice, you close the distance between the way you want to live and the lifestyle you want to leave behind.
—Jenny Craig

If you can think of yourself as creator of your life, take a moment to look at the conditions you've attracted into it. This may mean spending a little time each day alone, away from the hustle and bustle. Recording your thoughts and observations in a journal can help you to gain insight. Ask yourself: "What is my current health status?"

Can you see any connection between your thoughts/feelings/ actions and your health status? Do you see any room for adjustments that might lead you to an entirely new state of health?

Persevere

We all have dreams. But in order to make dreams into reality, it takes an awful lot of determination, dedication, self-discipline, and effort.
—Jesse Owens

We were playing a friendly game of "Gender Gap™" one night with some friends. One of the questions in this popular board game asked: "What is the most important character trait for success?" The answer wasn't your physical attractiveness, networking ability, or your choice of careers. It was *gumption!* Successful people take the initiative to get going and have the perseverance to keep going—no matter what! They do not give up at the first sign of rejection or the first "No" or even the tenth "No!" They commit themselves to continual improvement and see each setback as a learning opportunity for future endeavors.

Health Miracle Activities

1. Create a gratitude list for yourself. What are some of the things that you are grateful for? Keep this list near your bed so that you can read it each morning and night.

   _____
   _____
   _____

2. What negative thoughts and feelings have been blocking you from achieving the health that you deserve?

   _____
   _____

3. What is your desire for your health?

   _____
   _____

4. Visualize yourself already having the results of achieving your desired health. See it, smell it, taste it, feel it!

5. Make yourself a vision board. Cut pictures out of magazines, put photos of yourself among the pictures—have some fun with it! Stand back and experience marvelous results in due time.

Chapter 14

If you want to be happy, set a goal that commands your thoughts, liberates your energy, and inspires your hopes.
— Andrew Carnegie

The Miracle of Goal Setting

If you limit your choices only to what seems possible or reasonable, you discon-nect yourself from what you truly want, and all that is left is a compromise.
—Robert Fritz

We spent 10 years researching the information in this book and one of the most memorable experiences was being mentored by Mark Victor Hansen (coauthor of *Chicken Soup for the Soul*) and Robert Allen (author of *One-Minute Millionaire*). These gentlemen have spent the greater part of their lives studying success, goal setting, and acting on your dreams.

Kary's Story

One of our first dates back in 1998 was a Mark Victor Hansen live event. At the end of his inspirational talk, Mark challenged the entire audience to go home and write out 100 goals. He reported that only 2 percent of any of his audiences complete the task. Not wanting to fall in the trap of being part of the majority who don't, we made a commitment to be part of the few who do.

Uche invited me home to complete the task. Looking back, I realize he might have had ulterior motives! We were inspired and determined to take action, so we did just that! Uche got out some beautiful paper and put on some great music and we started to write our lists. About 45 minutes and 100 goals later, we were exhausted and uplifted. It felt good to write what I sometimes dared to dream about,

(continued)

such as writing a book one day, or modeling in a fitness magazine, or competing at the Olympia, or meeting Arnold Schwarzenegger, or speaking to thousands of people all over the world.

At the time of writing this book, I fondly look back at that first of many lists and sometimes experience utter amazement that I have checkmarks beside 50 of the goals I wrote 10 years ago! I did write a book, model in fitness magazines, compete at the Olympia, and meet Arnold Schwarzenegger!

What Are Goals?

People don't fail because they aim too high and miss, but because they aim too low and hit.

—Les Brown

A goal is simply a dream with a deadline. Everyone has dreams, but not everyone sets the goals that make the dreams a reality. The process of goal setting is essential to a successful life. The benefits are plentiful. The pursuit of a goal adds life to your days. The journey becomes more enjoyable. Goals energize and enliven you and motivate you to leap out of bed in the morning! The process of goal setting helps you to break down your dreams into attainable steps. Just ask any successful person about the importance of goal setting.

Champions in every field consistently do the things that average people choose not to do—like setting specific goals. Baseball great Lou Vickery shared an insight: "Four short words sum up what has lifted most successful individuals above the crowd: a little bit more. They did all that was expected of them and a little bit more."

Health Miracle

A great speaker once encouraged a university class to write out their goals. The university decided to study the outcomes of this challenge. They surveyed the class and found that only 3 percent had written out goals for their lives. Ten years later, they interviewed the participants and found that the 3 percent with written goals had achieved more in their lives than the other 97 percent!

What's Holding You Back?

A man too busy to take care of his health is like a mechanic too busy to take care of his tools.
—Spanish proverb

Okay, so you've heard it all before. Maybe you have even tried writing down some goals, and you're feeling a little disheartened. The challenge you may be facing—even if you've experienced some success and have achieved some of your goals—is that you have stopped setting them. Or you haven't dared to set them high enough.

When you were in your teens, did you think that you would end up looking or feeling like you do today? Imagine if you went back to that time in your life and had the opportunity to do it all over again. Would you do it differently? It reminds one of what baseball legend Mickey Mantle once said: "If I knew I was going to live this long, I'd have taken better care of myself."

Be honest. Lately, have you sat down and done some real dreaming, leaving your limitations and circumstances out of the picture? Or has one of the following complaints held you back:

I Can't Get Started
Beginning is half the battle in any project. Earl Nightingale said, "The majority of people who have failed are people who never began." With respect to health and wellness, most people have only a vague idea of what they want. Top athletes are usually the only ones who have set health and performance goals for themselves. Most people, if they set any goals, may have done it for their careers, but not for their health. This is one of the reason why 67 percent of Americans and 59 percent of Canadians are overweight. We encourage you to think back to your powerful reasons for acting on your health. And just think of all the health miracles you have read about in this book. It's time for you to *take action* and enjoy the results you deserve!

I Don't Believe It Will Work
Doubt will trip up even the best of us at some point in our lives. Don't worry, you are not alone. Shakespeare wrote, "Our doubts are traitors, and make us lose the good we oft might win by fearing to attempt." Sometimes you have to suspend your doubts and trust that the experts know what they are talking about! If you needed absolute proof for

everything that happens in your life, you would be a basket case! After all, we get on a plane without ever seeing the pilot, yet we trust that he or she is there. At least writing out goals can't kill you. Suspend your disbelief for a few minutes and play along.

I Do Urgent Versus Essential Tasks

Stephen Covey, in *Seven Habits of Highly Effective People*, says that the tragedy of our modern-day society is that people spend most of their time on the urgent day-to-day tasks, caught up in a daily schedule. The lawn needs mowing, you need groceries, the kids need new school supplies, you have to go to work, and then you need to get ready to do it all over again. This leaves little time for essential, but non-urgent activities like dreaming, goal setting, or exercising. Successful people in all areas of life make more time for these activities.

I Am Scared of Failing

Anytime we have asked people in our seminars why they haven't written down their goals, we get a response like: "Why set myself up for failure?" We say: "Why set yourself up to say 'I wish I had. . . .'" Now that would be a tragedy. Norman Cousins said, "Death is not the greatest loss in life. The greatest loss is what dies inside us while we live." Having a 100-goal list can alleviate your fear of failure. On that list you will have several easy, attainable goals along with your big, spectacular dreams. The small easy goals will inspire you and will create forward momentum and a sense of achievement. Your goal list is not static—you can review it as often as you like, you can stroke off things that no longer matter to you—it's your list! And having many goals means that you will eventually have many checkmarks. Maybe you won't achieve everything in your lifetime, but at least you will achieve *something*!

Design Your Best Life

The best way to succeed in the future is to create it.
   —Robin Sharma

In life, we all want good things to happen to us. The challenge is that most of us usually have only a vague idea of what we truly want. How are you supposed to shoot an arrow and hit a target that is not there? Can you imagine a sports team setting foot on a field without a game plan?

Do you believe you could have the body or health you truly desire if you had more *power?* Power is what goal setting will give you. It is one of the best ways to utilize the awesome forces in your mind. Most people only utilize 5–10 percent of their brains' potential.

David's Story

After reading your book and attending your seminar, I was inspired to make some changes in my life. My fiftieth birthday came and went last October. My midline was gradually expanding and I was feeling moderately tired a lot of the time. I enlisted the help of a personal trainer at a gym and decided to be more fastidious in adhering to healthy eating habits. My goals were:

- *do muscle training twice a week*
- *play squash twice a week*
- *do one flexible hour a week of light aerobic activity at home*
- *have two rest days a week*
- *eat three healthy meals with snacks in between*
- *get out of the kitchen after dinner*
- *cave in to cravings occasionally*
- *eat organic foods when possible*
- *use the stairs when possible*

The results have been a waist reduction from 36 inches to 32 inches, some weight loss, increased upper body mass, marked increase in general energy level, less backache, and I think a better disposition toward family, staff, and friends.

A Shift in Consciousness

A man's mind stretched to a new idea never goes back to its original dimensions.
   —Oliver Wendell Holmes

Goal setting is the place to start. It is the master key to achieving the level of health and fitness you want and deserve. Goal setting helps you concentrate your energy and power. It gives you self-confidence and provides enthusiasm for when events don't go exactly as planned. Goals also inspire you to become more decisive; you will see much more clearly the direction you need to go. And miraculously, opportunities will become available. Just by reading *The Miracle of Health* you will find that your awareness has shifted.

How does goal setting come into play with your health? Instead of saying, "I want to lose a few pounds." You will now say, "I want to lose 10 pounds over six months using sound nutrition principles, weight training, power walking, and yoga."

Your unconscious mind is your true power center. Most people rarely access this part of their brain. It stores all information and never sleeps. It is busy 24 hours a day, working out solutions long after problems have been dumped there by the conscious mind. Your unconscious mind works with pictures and visual images, so by writing down your goals and visualizing them, you can put your unconscious mind to work for you. Now *that* is the miracle of goal setting!

It was one of our goals to become sought-after speakers on health and wellness. This goal aroused a lot of emotion in us. We are passionate about sharing the benefits of excellent nutrition and physical activity! We once read that our unconscious mind works with pictures, so we pasted a picture of ourselves on a magazine cover under the headline: The Top 100 Lecturers. We then taped it to the bathroom mirror. This was in 2005. One day in 2008, we looked at our speaking schedule for 2009 on the big calendar in our home office and realized that our calendar was quickly filling up with speaking engagements at some of the most prestigious professional-development programs in North America! Once again, the power of goal setting at work.

Health Miracle

One of the top New Year's goals is to quit smoking. Christine Northrup, M.D., *New York Times* best-selling author, said that more people die from smoking-related diseases than from car accidents, suicides, cocaine, heroin, and alcoholism *combined*! Benefits to quitting occur immediately. Did you know that 24 hours after a person stops smoking, the risk for a heart attack decreases; after two to three weeks, lung function rises up to 30 percent; and after one to nine months, coughing and fatigue decrease?

Painful Consequences

Never have to say: "I wish I had . . ."
　—Kary Odiatu

Before we ask you to write down some of your own goals for your health, imagine your life and your future if you do not make any changes to the way you are thinking, acting, and living right now. This is a tough exercise. Dig deep and expose in detail any consequences you will experience if you do not change your current habits and start to realize your ideal health and fitness plan. What will you think and feel about yourself if you do not make it happen? Who would be affected if you do not take care of your physical self? What kind of role model would you be? What kind of legacy will you leave? How will your children and grandchildren remember you?

Do not write these thoughts down—remember, there is power in the written word. The only reason we even ask you to think like this is because sometimes it takes a little pain to spur you into action. We have come to the end of our book and if all of the health miracles in this book have not already inspired you to take action, then we have to pull out all the stops!

Let's turn the tables now and get your conscious and unconscious minds working for you.

Identifying Your Health Goals

Dreams move us beyond what we believe is realistic. And what we believe is realistic holds us back, limits us, to what we can achieve.
　—Silken Laumann

Now it's time to write down at least 10 specific goals in the areas of health and wellness. For example, your ideal percentage of body fat; a strength goal (e.g., "I will perform 10 push-ups"); a new sport you would like to try (e.g., rock climbing); the number of hours per week you would like to spend on fitness; your ideal weight; an activity you would love to do with your family; a target resting heart rate (say, 65 beats a minute); becoming a nonsmoker; drinking eight glasses of water every day; eating at least one more serving of fruits and vegetables, starting some fish oil supplements today; walking 1 mile every day—you get the idea.

Write them down as if you already do the activity or have accomplished the feat. Begin with the words, "I am" or "I have." The idea is to train your mind to see yourself already achieving the goal. Remember that the mind cannot tell the difference between an intensely imagined event and a real one.

As you're setting your goals, it is important to act as if failure is impossible or not even an issue. Before you start, we ask that you put yourself in a state of total certainty. Remember when you were a child and it was the night before your birthday or the night before Christmas? You could barely sleep because you knew that the next day would be filled with great joy.

If you have some music that really motivates you, use it to heighten your state of total certainty. With your music in the background, breathe deeply and really feel all that bound-up energy in your body. Close your eyes for a minute and breathe deeply. Picture all the wonderful health- and fitness-related dreams you desire for yourself. Once you feel certain, nod to yourself and begin writing quickly.

1. _____

2. _____

3. _____

4. _____

5. _____

6. _____

7. _____

8. _____

9. _____

10. _____

Now, beside each of your goals, write a deadline for its achievement. If you only have goals that will take longer than one year to accomplish, then you need to come up with some short-term, smaller goals you can accomplish within the next year. Short-term goals lead you toward your long-term goal(s). For example, if your long-term goal is to run a marathon next year, then you can come up with several short-term goals toward its achievement (i.e., invest in a new pair of running shoes, join a running club, subscribe to *Runner's Magazine*, read a book about marathon training, etc.). You can see how your goal list can become quite long! Some of the goals will be more challenging to reach, and others will be easy. It is these smaller accomplishments that will lead you daily toward the long-term goals and keep your motivation strong.

Remember that this is your list and you can review it at will. Goals and dates can be revised or stroked off your list. The more goals you have, the more checkmarks you will see at the end of the year, and the more successful you will feel!

Benefits and Reasons

Everyone wants to be strong and self-sufficient, but few are willing to put in the work necessary to achieve these goals.
—Gandhi

Pick out one or two of your very important long-term goals. Write one paragraph for each goal, describing in detail the benefits you will enjoy as you work toward this goal. These are the reasons. Reasons are the power behind the dream. This will help you to connect powerful feelings to the achievement of your dream. Don't worry about how it will happen at this point. The key is to anchor strong and empowering reasons and feelings that will propel you forward.

If your goal is to run in the Boston Marathon and you live in Moose Jaw, Canada, it's more important to know *why* you want to run than *how* you're going to get there. As long as your *why* is powerful enough, the *how* will appear.

Jack Canfield tells a story in his book, *The Success Principles*, about Olympic athlete Dan O'Brien. He was one of many athletes preparing to compete in the toughest event at the summer Olympics. The decathlon is a grueling 10-event competition where the winner gets the title of the "World's Greatest Athlete." Dan O'Brien was the only athlete in a room full of Olympic hopefuls who raised his hand when Bruce Jenner (1976 Olympic decathlon gold medalist) asked if anyone in the room had their list of goals with them at that moment. Later that week, Dan O'Brien won the gold medal at the 1996 Olympics in Atlanta!

Take Action

You can't hire other people to do your push-ups for you!
    —Jim Rohn

Did you take the required action and write down your goals? Just reading this chapter will not get you closer to looking and feeling good. If you completed all the exercises, congratulations! You are well on your way. Even if you wrote only one goal, it could be the one that kick-starts your health quest.

Uche's Story

> *Every year I take my top five goals from my 100 list and write them on an index card that I carry with my in my wallet. Whenever I reach in my wallet for a credit card or money, I see my list and I am reminded of my personal commitment to live my life on purpose with these goals. It's my own private pick-me-up.*

Once you make the decision to move toward health and vitality, it's extremely important to take immediate action to let the universe know you're serious. As soon as you say to yourself that enough is enough—that you're sick and tired of being sick and tired—that's the time to make a phone call to your doctor's office for a complete physical. That's the time to go to your kitchen and start clearing out all the junk food from the deepest, darkest depths of your cupboards. Concrete action steps taken with conviction bring you closer to your goals. And the only way to keep the fire of desire alive is to fan the flames with purposeful action! Jean-Jacques Rousseau once said, "To live is not merely to breathe, it is to act; it is to make use of our organs, senses, faculties. . . ." There must be one action step, one of your short-term goals, that you can act on today to show that you mean business. As author Henry James once said, "It's time to start living the life you've imagined!"

There are only two ways to live your life. One is as though nothing is a miracle. The other is as though everything is a miracle.
    —Albert Einstein

Bibliography

Anderson, Dr. James W., and Dr. Maury M. Breecher. *Dr. Anderson's Antioxidant, Anti-aging Health Program.* New York: Carroll & Graf, 1996.

Applegate, Liz. *Encyclopedia of Sports and Fitness Nutrition.* New York: Three Rivers Press, 2002.

Arntz, William, B. Chasse, and M. Vicente. *What the Bleep Do We Know!?* Deerfield Beach: Health Communications, 2005.

Augustine, Sue. *With Wings There Are No Barriers.* Gretna: Pelican Publishing Company, 1996.

Birch, L.L., S.L. Johnson, G. Andresen, J.S. Peters, and M.C. Schulte. "The Variability of Young Children's Energy Intake." *New England Journal of Medicine* 324 (1991):232.

Brooks, Douglas. *Effective Strength Training.* Champaign: Human Kinetics, 2001.

Buscaglia, Leo. *Born for Love.* Thorofare: SLACK Incorporated, 1992.

_____. *Living, Loving & Learning.* New York: Ballantine Books, 1982.

Byrne, Rhonda. *The Secret.* Hillsboro: Beyond Words Publishing, 2006.

Canfield, Jack. *The Success Principles.* New York: HarperCollins, 2005.

Chek, Paul. *Eat Move and Be Healthy.* San Diego: C.H.E.K. Institute, 2004.

Chopra, Dr. Deepak. *Magical Mind, Magical Body.* Niles: Nightingale-Conant Corporation, 1990.

_____. *Seven Spiritual Laws of Success.* San Rafael: Amber-Allen Publishing, 1995.

Coehlo, Paulo. *The Alchemist.* New York: HarperCollins, 1993.

Colbin, Annemarie. *Food and Healing.* New York: Ballantine Books, 1986.

Colcombe, S.J., et al. "Aerobic Fitness Reduces Brain Tissue Loss in Aging Humans." *The Journals of Gerontology, Series A: Biological Science and Medical Sciences* 58 (2003):M176–M180.

Cousins, Dr. Norman. *Anatomy of an Illness.* New York: Norton, 2001.

_____. *Head First: The Biology of Hope.* Toronto: Penguin Books, 1989.

Covey, Steven. *Seven Habits of Highly Effective People* New York: Simon & Schuster, 1989.

_____. *The Quest.* New York: Simon & Schuster, 1996.

_____, and Sandra Merrill Covey. *Seven Habits of Highly Effective Families.* New York: Golden Books, 1997.

Craig, Jenny. *Jenny Craig's Little Survival Guide.* Des Moines: Oxmoor House, 1996.

Crenshaw, L. *The Alchemy of Love and Lust.* New York: Pocket Books, 1997.

Crowley, C., and H. Lodge. *Younger Next Year: A Guide to Living Like 50 Until You're 80 and Beyond.* New York: Workman Publishing Co., 2004.

D'Adamo, Dr. Peter J. *Cook Right 4 Your Type.* New York: Berkley Books, 1999.

Dass, Ram. *Journey of Awakening.* New York: Bantam Books, 1990.

Demartini, Dr. John. *You Can Have an Amazing Life in Just 60 Days!* Carlsbad: Hay House, 2005.

Dennis, K.E. "Weight Management in Women." *Nursing Clinics of North America* 39 (2004):231–241.

Dollemore, Doug, and Mark Giuliucci. *Age Erasers for Men.* New York: St. Martin's Press, 1997.

Dyer, Dr. Wayne. *Being in Balance.* Carlsbad: Hay House Publishing, 2006.

_____. *Inspiration.* Carlsbad: Hay House Publishing, 2006.

_____. *Manifest Your Destiny.* Niles: Nightingale Conant, 1996.

_____. *Power of Intention.* Carlsbad: Hay House, 2004.

Eker, T. Harv. *Secrets of the Millionaire Mind.* New York: Harper Collins, 2005.

Fletcher, Anne M. *Eating Thin for Life.* Shelburne: Chapters Publishing Ltd., 1994.

Fulford, Dr. Robert C. *Dr. Fulford's Touch of Life.* New York: Pocket Books, 1997.

Gawain, Shakti. *Living in the Light.* Novato: Nataraj Publishing, 1998.

Godek, Greg. *Love: The Course They Forgot to Teach You in School.* Naperville: Sourcebooks Casablanca Press, 1997.

Graci, Sam. *The Food Connection.* Toronto: Macmillan Canada, 2001.

Graci, Sam. *The Path to Phenomenal Health.* Toronto: John Wiley & Sons, 2005.

_____, Dr. Carolyn DeMarco, and Dr. Letitia Rao. *The Bone-Building Solution.* Toronto: John Wiley & Sons, 2006.

Gray, John. *The Mars and Venus Diet and Exercise Solution.* New York: St. Martin's Press, 2003.

Grieger, J.A., et al. "Multivitamin Supplementation Improves Nutritional Status and Bone Quality in Aged Care Residents." *European Journal of Clinical Nutrition.* Online publication (November 28, 2007).

Hakala, Dee. *Thin Is Just a Four-Letter Word.* New York: Little, Brown and Company, 1997.

Hawkings, David. *Power versus Force.* Carlsbad: Hay House, 2002.

Hay, Louise. *You Can Heal Your Life.* Carlsbad: Hay House, 1999.

Hicks, Esther, and Jerry. *The Law of Attraction.* Carlsbad: Hay House, 2006.

Holtz, Lou. *Winning Every Day.* New York: HarperCollins, 1998.

Izzo, John. *The Five Secrets You Must Discover Before You Die.* San Francisco: Berrett-Koehler Publications Inc., 2008.

Kabat-Zinn, Jon. *Wherever You Go There You Are.* New York: Hyperion, 2005.

King, Brad J. *Fat Wars.* Toronto: Macmillan Canada, 2000.

Lamm, Dr. Steven. *Younger at Last.* New York: Simon & Schuster, 1997.

MacLaine, Shirley. *The Camino*. New York: Pocket Books, 2000.

_____. *Going Within*. New York: Bantam Doubleday Dell Publishing, 1989.

Maltz, Maxwell. *Psycho Cybernetics*. Englewood Cliffs: Prentice-Hall, 1960.

Masley, Dr. Steven. *Ten Years Younger*. New York: Broadway, 2007.

McGuire, D.K., et al. "Effect of Age on Cardiovascular Adaptation to Exercise Training." *Circulation* 104 (2001):1358–1366.

Monaghan, Dan, and Paul Monaghan. *Why Not Me?* New York: Prime Books Inc., 1992.

Naisbitt, John, and Patricia Aburdene. *Megatrends 2000*. New York: Avon Books, 1990.

Northrup, Dr. Christiane. *Mother-Daughter Wisdom*. New York: Bantam, 2005.

O'Brien, Dr. Mary. *Successful Aging*. Concord: Biomed Books, 2007.

Oz, Dr. Mehmet, and Dr. Michael Roizen. *You: The Owner's Manual*. New York: HarperCollins, 2005.

_____, and Dr. Michael Roizen. *You: Staying Young*. New York: Free Press, 2007.

Patchell-Evans, David. *Living the Good Life*. Toronto: ECW Press, 2004.

Pausch, Randy. *The Last Lecture*. New York: Hyperion, 2008.

Pearsall, Paul. *Making Miracles*. Englewood Cliffs: Prentice Hall Press, 1991.

_____. *Ten Laws of Lasting Love*. New York: Simon & Schuster, 1993.

Perls, Dr. Thomas T., and Margery H. Silver. *Living to 100: Lessons in Living to Your Maximum Potential at Any Age.* Jackson: Basic Books, 2000.

Pert, Candace. *Molecules of Emotion.* New York: Touchstone, 1999.

Peterson, Wilfred. *The Art of Living.* New York: Avon Books, 1990.

Phillips, Bill. *Body for Life.* New York: HarperCollins, 1999.

Phillips, Bill. *Eating for Life.* Golden: High Point Media, 2003.

Popcorn, Faith, and Lys Marigold. *Clicking: 16 Trends to Future Fit Your Life, Your Work, and Your Business.* New York: HarperCollins, 1996.

Powter, Susan. *Food.* New York: Simon & Schuster, 1995.

Proctor, Bob. *Born Rich.* Scottsdale: Life Success Productions, 2002.

Ratey, Dr. John. *Spark.* New York: Little, Brown and Company, 2008.

Ray, James Arthur. *Harmonic Wealth.* New York: Hyperion, 2008.

Ray, James Arthur. *The Science of Success.* Carlsbad: SunArk Press, 2006.

Redfield, James. *Celestine Prophecy.* Clayton: Warner Books, 1993.

_____. *Celestine Vision.* Clayton: Warner Books, 1999.

Ringer, Robert. *Million-Dollar Habits.* New York: Fawcett, 1990.

Rippe, Dr. James M. *Fit for Success.* Englewood Cliffs: Prentice Hall, 1989.

Robbins, Anthony. *Awaken the Giant within.* New York: Simon & Schuster, 1991.

Roger, John, and Peter McWilliams. *Wealth 101.* Santa Monica: Prelude Press, 1992.

Rona, Dr. Zoltan P. *Return to the Joy of Health*. Vancouver: Alive Books, 1995.

Ruiz, Don M. *The Four Agreements*. San Rafael: Amber-Allen Publishing, 1997.

St. James, Elaine. *Living the Simple Life*. New York: Hyperion, 1996.

Schucman, H. and W. Thetford, *A Course in Miracles*, Mill Valley: Foundation for Inner Peace, 2007.

Schwartz, David J. *The Magic of Thinking Big*. Englewood Cliffs: Prentice-Hall, 1965.

Seligman, Martin. *Learned Optimism*. New York: Free Press, 1998.

Sharma, Robin S. *Family Wisdom from the Monk Who Sold His Ferrari*. New York: Harper Collins, 2001.

_____. *The Monk Who Sold His Ferrari*. New York: HarperCollins, 1997.

Shiina, Y., et al. "Acute Effect of Oral Flavanoid-Rich Dark Chocolate Intake on Coronary Circulation." *International Journal of Cardiology* (November 26, 2007).

Shubentsov, Yefim. *Cure Your Cravings*. New York: G.P. Putnam's Sons, 1998.

Shulman, Dr. Joey. *The Last 15: A Weight-Loss Breakthrough*. Toronto: John Wiley & Sons, 2008.

_____. *The Natural Makeover Diet*. Toronto: John Wiley & Sons, 2005.

Thorne, Gerard, and Phil Embleton. *BODYFitness for Women*. Toronto: Musclemag International, 1999.

Timberlake, Lewis. *Born to Win*. Carol Stream: Tyndale House, 1986.

Tribole, Evelyn, and Elyse Resch. *Intuitive Eating: A Recovery Book for the Chronic Dieter.* New York: St. Martin's Press, 1995.

Tolle, Eckhart. *The New Earth.* New York, Penguin, 2005.

Tolle, Eckhart. *The Power of Now.* Novato: New World Libraries, 1999.

Waitley, Dennis. *The Double Win.* New York: Berkley Publishing Group, 1986.

Waldman, Mark R. *The Art of Staying Together.* New York: Tarcher, 1998.

Wansink, Brian. *Mindless Eating.* New York: Bantam Dell, 2006.

Weil, Dr. Andrew. *Healthy Aging.* New York: Alfred A. Knopf, 2005.

Willcox, Bradley J., et al. *The Okinawa Program.* New York: Three Rivers Press, 2001.

Williamson, Marianne. *The Age of Miracles: Embracing the New Midlife.* Carlsbad: Hay House, 2008.

Wright, Judith. *The One Decision.* New York: Tarcher, 2005.

Ziglar, Zig. *Over the Top.* Nashville: Thomas Nelson Publishers, 1994.